DIET

— AND —

EXERCISE
DIARY

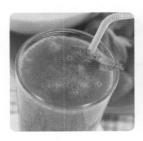
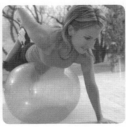
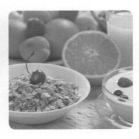

hinkler

Published by Hinkler Books Pty Ltd
45–55 Fairchild Street
Heatherton Victoria 3202 Australia
www.hinkler.com.au

hinkler

© Hinkler Books Pty Ltd 2007, 2011

Cover design: Hinkler Design Studio
Prepress: Graphic Print Group

ISBN:978 1 7430 8780 0

Printed and bound in China

Image Credits:
Images © Shutterstock.com: Woman stretching © Dmitriy Shironosov; Healthy
breakfast © Magone. Istock.com: Biceps © nico_blue; Pasta meal © Maica; Fruit
drink © og-vision.Woman on ball: Ned Meldrum

INTRODUCTION

We'd all love to be fit and healthy with no effort. Unfortunately, it can take a lot of hard work to achieve your fitness and weight loss goals. The *Diet and Exercise Diary* is a great tool to make it easier to reach those objectives.

By recording your dietary and exercise habits, you'll become more aware of what you put in your body and what you need to do to burn it off. With this knowledge comes a better understanding of how your actions affect your body. Use this information to set goals and targets, plan your diet and exercise sessions and gain a greater awareness of what works for you.

Remember, if you are starting a new diet or exercise regime, it is a good idea to have a check-up with your doctor first.

HEALTH AND WEIGHT

While most people would like to be slim for aesthetic reasons, there are other, more serious reasons for maintaining a healthy weight. It is well known that health experts are becoming increasingly concerned with the number of people who are overweight or obese.

The World Health Organization (WHO) has stated that at least one in three adults are overweight and one in 10 are obese. Someone who is even slightly overweight has an increased risk of health problems, and this risk increases the more overweight a person becomes. Carrying extra weight increases the chance of heart disease, stroke, diabetes, osteoarthritis, cancer, skin problems, respiratory conditions, infertility, gallbladder disease and hypertension.

The body mass index (BMI) is an easy way to measure whether someone is considered overweight. To obtain your BMI, use the following formula:

BMI = weight in kilograms divided by the square of height in metres

A woman who weighs 76 kg and is 1.79 m tall works out her BMI by dividing 76 by 3.2 (her height of 1.79 squared, or 1.79 x 1.79). 76 divided by 3.2 equals a BMI of 23.75.

The classifications used by the WHO are listed below.

Classification	BMI
Underweight	← 18.50
Healthy range	18.50–24.99
Overweight	25.00–29.99
Obese	30.00–39.99
Morbidly obese	→ 40.00

A person's body shape, build and ethnic origin can affect their BMI, so the figure is to be used as a guide only. People from an Asian background are classified as overweight if their BMI is greater than 23 and people with a Pacific Islander background are classified as overweight if their BMI is greater than 26. The BMI shouldn't be used for children under 15 or the elderly.

The health risks are found to be even greater if a person is carrying excess fat around their abdomen (such as a pot or beer belly). If your BMI is over 25 and your waist measurement is greater than 94 cm (37 in) for men and 80 cm (31.5 in) for women, your risk of disease is greater than a person who gains weight on other parts of their body, such as their arms, thighs and hips.

However, it's not all bad news! While excess weight can cause all sorts of health problems, it's also something that is well within your power to control. While your genetic makeup can influence your weight, balancing your calorie intake and your physical activity is the best way to lose weight. By making changes to your diet and lifestyle, you'll not only reduce your risk of disease, you'll also feel happier, have more energy, sleep better, handle stress more effectively and look great!

DIET
The modern diet is often made up of refined foods high in saturated fats and sugar and low in fibre, nutrients, vitamins and minerals. A healthy diet focuses on a variety of foods that provide the body with the right amount of fuel and nutrition it needs.

Read the labels on food packaging to get an idea of what nutrients, fat content and energy the food contains. An up-to-date fat, fibre and kilojoule/calorie counter is a great investment.

What foods should I eat?
A good diet is made up of foods that are high in fibre and low in fat.

Nutritionists recommend more:
- Vegetables (women: 4–7 serves per day; men: 6–8 serves per day)
- Fruit (women: 2–3 serves per day; men: 3–4 serves per day)
- Legumes and nuts (women: 1–1½ serves per day; men: 1–1½ serves per day)
- Wholegrain cereal, bread, rice, pasta and noodles (women: 4–6 serves per day; men: 5–7 serves per day)
- Lean meat and poultry (2–3 serves per week) and fish (1–2 per week)
- Water (at least a litre and a half of fluid or 3 pints per day, more in hot climates)

Nutritionists recommend less:
- Fat, especially saturated fats
- Sugar and sugary food and drinks
- Salt
- Alcohol (limit to one per day for women and two per day for men)

Kilojoules and calories
The body constantly needs to burn fuel to survive. Any excess fuel that is not burned by the body ends up being stored as excess fat. The energy found in foods is measured by kilojoules or calories.

The amount of carbohydrates, protein and fats found in food determine the number of kilojoules or calories that a food will have. Fat and alcohol have a lot more kilojoules or calories than carbohydrates, proteins and dietary fibre, therefore a high-fat diet encourages weight gain.

As an average, active women need around 5800–6700 kJ/1400–1600 calories a day, while sedentary women need around 4600–5400kJ/1100–1300 calories. Active men need about 7500–8400 kJ/1800–2000 calories per day and sedentary men need around 6700–7500 kJ/1600–1800 calories. These numbers are a guide only, and can vary depending on a person's build and metabolism.

Fat

Fat plays an important role in the body, so it is vital that a diet contains a little fat. It helps with hormone production, protects organs and assists the body absorb nutrients. However, there are different types of fat, some that raise blood cholesterol and others that lower it.

Avoid saturated fats (found in animal products such fatty meat and full fat dairy products, sweet biscuits and fried foods) and trans fatty acids (found in some margarines and spreads) as these fats raise cholesterol levels.

Monounsaturated fats (in canola or olive oil-based spreads, canola, olive and peanut oil, most nuts and avocado) and polyunsaturated fats can help lower blood cholesterol and should be eaten in moderation. The two types of polyunsaturated fats, omega-3 (in oily fish, canola and soy) and omega-6 (in safflower and sunflower oil, seeds and nuts), are thought to be especially beneficial in lowering cholesterol and reducing the chance of blood clots.

Protein

Proteins are made up of amino acids. The body uses proteins to create, repair and maintain cells, provide energy and to make hormones. It is recommended that adults daily eat 0.75 grams (0.03 oz) of protein per kilogram (2.2 lb) of their bodyweight and older adults daily eat 1 gram (0.04 oz) per kilogram (2.2 lb). Good protein-rich foods include lean meat and poultry, fish, low-fat dairy products, eggs, nuts and seeds, beans, pulses and lentils, soy foods and wheat grains.

Carbohydrates

Carbohydrates are the major source of fuel for our bodies. Major organs such as the brain and kidneys rely on carbohydrates to function and it is also used to metabolise fat.

The body breaks down carbohydrates into sugars, such as glucose. In response to the rise in sugar levels, insulin is produced to help move glucose from the bloodstream to cells, where it is burned as energy. Excess glucose is converted into glycogen, which is stored in the liver and released when the body's sugar levels drop. Some carbohydrates break down into glucose very quickly, while others break down a lot slower, meaning glucose is released into the blood over a longer period of time. It is important to include carbohydrates into a healthy diet. The body will break down muscle tissue to turn into glucose if it is not getting enough carbohydrates.

The Glycaemic Index (GI)

The GI measures food by how quickly its carbohydrates are turned into glucose. Carbohydrates that quickly break down into glucose (high GI foods) affect blood sugar levels much faster than those that break down slowly (low GI foods). Low blood sugar levels trigger hunger. As a result, a low-GI diet can reduce hunger levels and keep blood sugar levels stabilised.

A good low-GI diet will include wholegrain breads, oats, barley, bran, basmati or brown rice, wholemeal pastas, couscous, beans and lentils, soy foods, fruit, vegetables, low-fat dairy products, nuts and oily fish.

Fibre

Dietary fibre is found in plant foods such as fruit, vegetables, legumes and cereals. Fibre contains no nutrients or calories in itself, but is essential for keeping the digestive system healthy and regular. There are two types of fibre: soluble (found in fruits, vegetables, bran, oats, seeds, lentils and soy foods) and insoluble (found in wholegrain foods, the skins of vegetables and fruit, beans, brans, brown rice, nuts and seeds). Soluble fibre can help to lower blood cholesterol and glucose levels and insoluble fibre improves the digestive system. Fibre also reduces the risks of some cancers, diabetes, heart disease and bowel disease.

Increasing the amount of fibre, especially soluble fibre, helps with weight loss. Fibre provides the feeling of fullness and satisfaction. As it takes longer to pass through the digestive system, this feeling lasts a lot longer than with low-fibre foods and also keeps blood sugar levels at a stabilised level. Foods containing fibre also have more nutrients and are usually low in fat and sugar. As fibre absorbs water, it is important to drink lots of water on a high-fibre diet. Try to consume at least 30 grams (1 oz) of fibre per day.

Nutrients

Eating a balanced diet ensures that your body will get the right amount of nutrients and minerals. Eating some lean meat and fish will prevent iron and zinc deficiencies, and eating lean meat with plant foods can actually increase iron absorption from the vegetables. Low-fat dairy foods are excellent sources of calcium, which helps build strong bones and teeth. Cereals supply the body with vitamins B and E.

Water and fluids

The body cannot survive without water. A person can live for weeks without food, but only a few days without water. Around two thirds of the body is made up of water. Water regulates body temperature and is the major component in blood, sweat, urine, saliva, eyes and stomach acids. It keeps the skin looking younger, carries nutrients to cells and cushions joints.

Drink plenty of water and fluids to avoid dehydration. Six to eight glasses or a litre and half (3 pints) per day are recommended by nutritionists. Drink coffee, tea and fruit juice in moderation, as coffee and tea contain caffeine and juice contains kilojoules/calories.

Healthy dieting tips

- Reduce portion and serving sizes. However, increase the number of red, green and yellow vegetable servings. Try adding an extra vegetable to your meals.
- Plan your meals in advance.
- Read the labels on food products. Some foods labelled 'low fat' are very high in sugar or kilojoules/calories.
- Prepare healthy snacks, such as fruit, nuts or wholemeal crackers, ahead of time.

- Don't boil vegetables for too long, as they will lose their nutrients and flavour.
- Use herbs and spices to flavour food, rather than adding fatty sauces or salt.
- Choose wholemeal and wholegrain cereals over white and processed cereals.
- Eat lots of fibre – you'll feel fuller.
- Don't set unachievable weight-loss goals.
- Eat a high-fibre breakfast, such as bran, whole wheat or oat cereal, every day.

EXERCISE

The rise in obesity levels has occurred at the same time as the increase in labour-saving devices and desk-based jobs. It's no surprise that a lower rate of activity means a greater rate of weight gain. It is now understood that activity plays as equally an important role as diet in maintaining a healthy weight.

Exercise is also thought to prevent a range of diseases, such as heart disease, hypertension, diabetes, stroke, some cancers and osteoporosis. It is also thought to be helpful in combating depression and anxiety, as well as a good way of dealing with stress. It can also increase your metabolism.

Cardio-vascular exercise

There are many ways you can increase your activity and movement levels. The WHO recommends moderate daily physical activity for at least 30 minutes a day. This sort of exercise should make you breathe so that you can comfortably talk but not sing and make your heart beat faster. Moderate exercise can include things such as brisk walking, light weight training, cycling and mowing the lawn.

It is also helpful to have a few sessions of more vigorous exercise that run for at least 30 minutes three or four days a week. This should make you puff so that talking is very hard and you break into a sweat. It includes activities such as jogging, fast swimming, exercise classes, squash, singles tennis, power walking, team sports and fast cycling. The WHO recommends at least 150 minutes of moderate activity or 75 minutes of vigorous activity a week. For extra benefit, increase moderate activity to 300 minutes or vigorous activity to 150 minutes a week.

Strength training

Strength or resistance training is important to build muscle and bone density. It improves metabolic rate, muscle mass and endurance. This is especially important as you age, as older people's muscles lose strength. Strength or resistance training includes free weights, strength training machines, exercising with bands or tubes, and callisthenics (such as sit-ups, push-ups and pull-ups).

It is a good idea to complete two or three sessions a week of resistance or weight training of at least 20 minutes. Perform around ten exercises for a minimum of eight to twelve repetitions. The intensity and weight will vary depending on your strength and fitness levels. Give yourself at least one day's break between training sessions for your muscles to repair and recover.

Stretching and flexibility

Regular stretching helps keep your body flexible and prevent muscle injury and soreness during exercise. It improves muscle elasticity by increasing blood flow to the muscles and helps lengthen and strengthen them. Never hold your breath as you stretch. Try and perform a range of long, slow stretches that target different muscles one by one. Yoga and tai chi are great activities that improve flexibility and also help you to relax.

Warming up and cooling down

Warming up before exercise involves slowly building up activity so that blood flow to the muscles increases and warms the tissues and the heart rate slowly increases. It also causes adrenalin to be released and lubricates the joints. A warm-up should relate to the exercise that you're about to perform. For example, if you were going to exercise your legs, you would do some gentle jogging on the spot. Some gentle stretches should also be performed.

Cooling down can help delay and reduce muscle soreness and should be done at a lower intensity than the main exercise. It keeps the blood flowing through the muscles, prevents the build up of lactic acid and prevents dizziness. Slowly reducing the rate of exercise for five to ten minutes and performing a series of stretches will help.

Incidental exercise

Increasing your activity in your daily life also plays an important part in weight loss. Incidental exercise is general activity that you do in your everyday life. It includes things such as walking to the bus, housework, taking the stairs and standing to change the television channel. This sort of exercise is thought to be very important to how much energy is expended each day. Look at your daily habits and see where you can incorporate more incidental exercise. Walk to a colleague's desk instead of phoning or emailing. Park the car as far from the door at the shops and walk.

Setting goals and staying motivated

It is important to make time for exercise. Set goals that are challenging but achievable, as you're bound to lose motivation if you keep failing to reach your targets. If necessary, talk to a fitness professional or research what sort of targets are appropriate for you and your level of fitness. Competing against yourself is a great way to get results. Try and beat your previous time or perform more repetitions. Look for handy gadgets such as pedometers, heart rate monitors and distance monitors that can help you record your performance.

It is easy to lose motivation if you try and achieve too much or if you're doing activities that you don't enjoy or that don't fit in with your lifestyle. Choose a variety of activities so that you won't get bored or frustrated easily. Exercising with a friend or with a trainer is a great way to keep motivated. Of course, there's no better motivation than reaching your goals and seeing the results of your hard work!

Exercise and activity tips

* Try and be active every day.
* Regard activity as a bonus, not a bother.
* Look for ways to be active in your everyday life.
* Choose activities and exercises that you enjoy.
* Make exercise a regular part of your family and social life.

- Work out with an exercise partner.
- Join a gym or fitness club, get a personal trainer or play a team sport.
- Set goals and try and beat them.
- Train for an event or competition.
- Don't be unrealistic with your targets – you can injure yourself trying to meet them or lose motivation.
- Use an exercise journal (such as this one!).

Activity	Approx. kJ/cal burned per hour	Activity	Approx. kJ/cal burned per hour
Sleeping	230/55	Brisk walking	1750/420
Eating	355/85	Basketball	1750/420
Sitting	355/85	Aerobics	1885/450
Standing	420/100	Moderate cycling	1885/450
Driving	460/110	Jogging	2090/500
Housework	670/160	Digging	2090/500
Golf	1000/240	Fast swimming	2090/500
Callisthenics	1000/240	Cross trainer	2090/500
Slow cycling	1000/240	Hiking	2090/500
Slow walking	1000/240	Step class	2300/550
Gardening	1045/250	Rowing	2300/550
Ballroom dancing	1090/260	Power walking	2510/600
Walking	1170/280	Heavy weight training	2510/600
Slow swimming	1250/300	Exercise bike or fast cycling	2720/650
Raking garden	1465/350	Squash	2720/650
Tennis (singles)	1465/350	Skipping	2390/700
Rollerblading	1750/420	Running	2390/700
Vigorous dancing	1750/420		

HOW TO USE THE DIARY

The *Diet and Exercise Diary* is designed to be a complete record for you to detail your exercise, eating and health habits over the course of twelve months. Not only is an exercise and diet diary a great way to track and analyse your progress and achievements, it also allows you to set and achieve your goals. This diary is divided into days, weeks, months and a year, so that you can extensively monitor your exercise and dietary practices and behaviours. As the diary is not dated, you can start recording your information at any time of year.

Twelve-month planner

The diary starts off with a twelve-month planner that allows you to record events over the course of a year. Use this section to fill in major events and occurrences that could affect your exercise sessions and dietary habits throughout the year. These may include things such as holidays, family celebrations, birthdays, work events and conferences, a new job or medical appointments and issues.

Yearly assessments

The yearly assessments are a great way to record your details at the start and end of the twelve-month period covered by the diary. Fill out your information at the beginning of your program and use the first assessment page to set out weight-loss goals and exercise targets. There's even space to include a photograph of yourself.

The end of year assessment spread will show you just how far you have come over the course of twelve months. You'll be able to assess whether you've met or even surpassed the goals that you set at the start of the diary. Again, there's space for a photograph of the new, improved you!

Weekly records

The weekly records form the major part of the dairy. You can set weekly targets, plan your calorie intake and record your weight and body mass index (BMI) at the beginning and end of the week. There's also space to record lifestyle information, such as energy and stress levels, appetite, mood and sleeping habits. You can also jot down possible diet-busting occasions that you may encounter during the week.

Use the food diary to record your daily totals of fat, protein, carbohydrates, fibre and calories. There's space to record your hunger scale as well as your coffee, tea and fluid intake. Add up the totals to show your overall weekly food consumption and compare it against your goal from the start of the week.

The exercise diary allows you to enter your strength and cardio training sessions throughout the week. Record your target area, the equipment used, the number of sets and reps and the weight you've used in your strength training. You can also note down information such as your heart rate, the exercise intensity and the calories you've burnt in your cardio sessions. In addition, keep a record of any incidental exercise you might have done. This can include taking the stairs, mowing the lawn, vacuuming the house or playing with the kids.

Monthly summary

Use the monthly summary to set goals and to show your progress over the past month. Check your average daily calorie, fat, protein, carbohydrate and fibre consumption over the course of a month, as well as your average stress, energy, mood and appetite levels. Again, there's room for a photograph to show any changes. By assessing your weight, fitness and body measurements at the start of the month and comparing it against your results at the end of the month, you'll not only have a great idea of your progress but also be motivated to keep up the good work!

Yearly weight graph

The weight graph is a great visual way to track your progress over the course of twelve months. Each week, simply mark your weight on the graph. Draw a line between each point as the year progresses and you'll get a good idea of how you are doing with your program.

Personal bests

Record your best times and results in this section. Keep updating this chart with your progress and new bests, and utilise this information to assist with setting new goals and targets.

Don't be discouraged if you occasionally miss a session or eat the wrong food – move on and pick up where you left off. The most important thing is that you are aware of what you put in your body and how you burn it off. Once you are able to analyse your progress over time, you'll have an idea of what works best for you and achieve even better results.

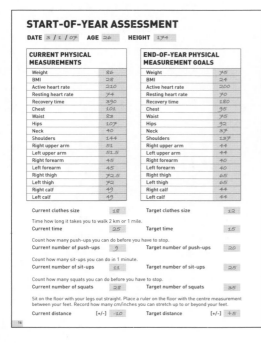

TWELVE-MONTH PLANNER

	JANUARY	FEBRUARY	MARCH	APRIL	MAY	JUNE
1						
2						
3						
4						
5						
6			Holiday			
7			↑			
8						
9				Work function		
10				Work function		
11	Dinner with Pete					
12						
13						
14			↓			
15	Day off		Holiday			
16						
17						
18						
19						
20						
21					Sarah's birthday	
22						
23	Ryan's birthday					
24						
25						
26						
27						
28						
29						
30						
31						
	JANUARY	FEBRUARY	MARCH	APRIL	MAY	JUNE

	JULY	AUGUST	SEPTEMBER	OCTOBER	NOVEMBER	DECEMBER	
							1
							2
							3
							4
							5
		W/end away					6
		W/end away					7
							8
			My birthday				9
							10
							11
							12
							13
							14
						Work break up	15
							16
							17
						Ryan's xmas party	18
							19
							20
							21
							22
							23
							24
						Christmas	25
							26
							27
							28
							29
							30
							31
	JULY	AUGUST	SEPTEMBER	OCTOBER	NOVEMBER	DECEMBER	

14

15

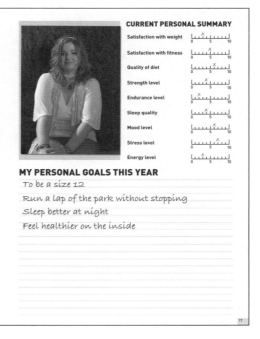

START-OF-YEAR ASSESSMENT

DATE 3 / 1 / 07   **AGE** 26   **HEIGHT** 174

CURRENT PHYSICAL MEASUREMENTS		END-OF-YEAR PHYSICAL MEASUREMENT GOALS	
Weight	86	Weight	75
BMI	28	BMI	24
Active heart rate	210	Active heart rate	200
Resting heart rate	74	Resting heart rate	70
Recovery time	390	Recovery time	180
Chest	101	Chest	95
Waist	83	Waist	75
Hips	107	Hips	92
Neck	40	Neck	37
Shoulders	144	Shoulders	137
Right upper arm	51	Right upper arm	44
Left upper arm	51.5	Left upper arm	44
Right forearm	45	Right forearm	40
Left forearm	45	Left forearm	40
Right thigh	72.5	Right thigh	65
Left thigh	72	Left thigh	65
Right calf	49	Right calf	44
Left calf	49	Left calf	44

Current clothes size	18	Target clothes size	12

Time how long it takes you to walk 2 km or 1 mile.

Current time	25	Target time	15

Count how many push-ups you can do before you have to stop.

Current number of push-ups	9	Target number of push-ups	20

Count how many sit-ups you can do in 1 minute.

Current number of sit-ups	11	Target number of sit-ups	25

Count how many squats you can do before you have to stop.

Current number of squats	28	Target number of squats	35

Sit on the floor with your legs out straight. Place a ruler on the floor with the centre measurement between your feet. Record how many cm/inches you can stretch up to or beyond your feet.

Current distance	[+/-] -10	Target distance	[+/-] +5

CURRENT PERSONAL SUMMARY

Satisfaction with weight	X at 4, scale 0–5–10
Satisfaction with fitness	X at 4
Quality of diet	X at 4
Strength level	X at 3
Endurance level	X at 3
Sleep quality	X at 4
Mood level	X at 6
Stress level	X at 6
Energy level	X at 3

MY PERSONAL GOALS THIS YEAR

To be a size 12

Run a lap of the park without stopping

Sleep better at night

Feel healthier on the inside

16

17

11

WEEK BEGINNING 12 / 2 / 07

Weight at start of week **82.5**
BMI at start of week **27**
Planned kJ/Cal this week **8400**
Possible diet-busting occasions this week
Dinner out Saturday night

Planned exercise sessions this week

	Exercise	Completed [Y/N]
Monday	Treadmill	Y
Tuesday	Swimming	N
Wednesday	Treadmill	Y
Thursday	Stepper	Y
Friday	Swimming	Y
Saturday	Stepper	N
Sunday	Treadmill	N

FOOD DIARY

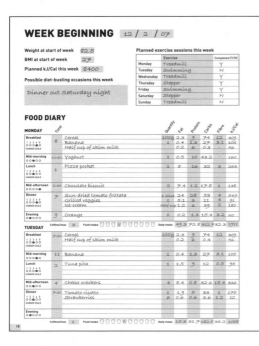

MONDAY

	Time		Quantity	Fat	Protein	Carbs	Fibre	kJ/Cal
Breakfast	8	Cereal	100g	23	9	74	12	309
		Banana	1	0.4	1.3	27	3.1	105
		Half cup of skim milk		0.2	6	0.3	-	56
Mid-morning	10:30	Yoghurt	1	0.5	10	43.2	-	160
Lunch	1	Pizza pocket	1	8	16	43	3	263
Mid-afternoon	2:30	Chocolate biscuit	2	7.4	1.2	17.8	1	138
Dinner	7	Sun-dried tomato frittata	1 slice	24	28	53	4	547
		Grilled veggies	1	5.1	3	11	4	91
		Ice-cream	half cup	1.2	6	39	2	180
Evening	9	Orange	1	0.2	1.3	15.4	3.2	60

Coffees/teas — Fluid intake — Daily totals **49.3 72.8 312 7 32.8 1911**

TUESDAY

	Time		Quantity	Fat	Protein	Carbs	Fibre	kJ/Cal
Breakfast	7:30	Cereal	100g	23	9	74	12	309
		Half cup of skim milk		0.2	6	0.3	-	56
Mid-morning	11	Banana	1	0.4	1.3	27	3.1	105
Lunch	2	Tuna pita	1	1.5	9	12	0.5	95
Mid-afternoon	4	Cheese crackers	4	24	0.8	32.6	18.4	336
Dinner	7:30	Tomato risotto	1	1.9	5	33	1	178
		Strawberries	8	0.6	0.6	3.6	1.2	12
Evening								

Coffees/teas 1 — Fluid intake — Daily totals **15.3 31.7 182.5 36.2 1088**

WEDNESDAY

	Time		Quantity	Fat	Protein	Carbs	Fibre	kJ/Cal
Breakfast	7:45	Scrambled eggs	1	24.4	21	16	3	362
Mid-morning	10	Apple muffin	1	3.7	4	24	3	139
Lunch	10:30	Vegetarian pizza	Slice	8	18	43	2	314
Mid-afternoon	3:30	Cheese roll	1	8	9	38	2	263
Dinner	6:30	Chicken stir-fry	1	4.4	27	6	2	175
Evening	9	Banana	1	0.4	1.3	27	3.1	105

Coffees/teas 0 — Fluid intake — Daily totals **48.9 80.3 154 15.1 1358**

THURSDAY

	Time		Quantity	Fat	Protein	Carbs	Fibre	kJ/Cal
Breakfast	7:30	Cereal	100g	23	9	74	12	309
		Half cup of skim milk		0.2	6	0.3	-	56
Mid-morning	10:45	Banana	1	0.4	1.3	27	3.1	105
Lunch	1	Mediterranean sub	1	10.5	22	72	5	470
Mid-afternoon	3:30	Raisin toast	2	17.6	10	62	4	434
Dinner	6	Pork and spinach stir-fry	1	13.9	21	5	2	227
		Ice-cream	half cup	1.2	6	39	2	180
Evening	8:30	Chocolate biscuit	2	7.4	1.2	17.8	1	138

Coffees/teas 1 — Fluid intake — Daily totals **53.5 102 237 6.1 28 1989**

FRIDAY

	Time		Quantity	Fat	Protein	Carbs	Fibre	kJ/Cal
Breakfast	8	Pancakes	1	4.8	4	16	1	123
		Blueberry sauce	1	0.2	-	11	2	46
Mid-morning	10	Orange	1	0.2	1.3	15.4	3.2	60
Lunch	12:30	Turkey wrap	1	13.4	22	59	7	428
Mid-afternoon	3:15	Diet jelly	1	-	1.1	5.2	0.1	13
Dinner	7	Spicy chicken	1	9.5	33	11	2	264
		Mediterranean veggies	1	4.7	1	6	1	67
Evening								

Coffees/teas 1 — Fluid intake — Daily totals **75.8 61.1 108.2 13.1 941**

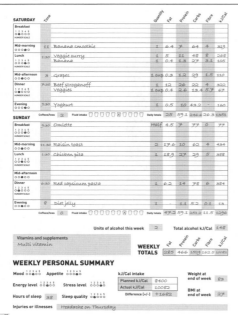

SATURDAY

	Time		Quantity	Fat	Protein	Carbs	Fibre	kJ/Cal
Breakfast								
Mid-morning	11	Banana smoothie	1	6.4	7	64	4	319
Lunch	1:30	Veggie curry	1	5	11	48	8	268
		Banana	1	0.4	1.3	27	3.1	105
Mid-afternoon	3	Grapes	1 cup	0.3	1.2	29	1.5	110
Dinner	7:30	Beef stroganoff	1	12	26	22	4	322
		Veggies	1 cup	0.4	2.6	13.4	5.7	67
Evening	9:30	Yoghurt	1	0.5	10	43.2	-	160

Coffees/teas 2 — Fluid intake — Daily totals **25 59.1 246.6 26.3 1351**

SUNDAY

	Time		Quantity	Fat	Protein	Carbs	Fibre	kJ/Cal
Breakfast	9:30	Omelette	Half	4.5	7	77	0	77
Mid-morning	11:30	Raisin toast	2	17.6	10	62	4	434
Lunch	1:30	Chicken pita	1	13.9	27	29	5	388
Mid-afternoon								
Dinner	6:30	Red capsicum pasta	1	6.2	14	78	6	384
Evening	8	Diet jelly	1	-	1.1	5.2	0.1	13

Coffees/teas — Fluid intake — Daily totals **47.2 59.1 251.2 11.5 1296**

Units of alcohol this week **2** — Total alcohol kJ/Cal **148**

Vitamins and supplements: *Multi vitamin*

WEEKLY TOTALS — Fat 285 — Protein 466 — Carbs 1529 — Fibre 162.5 — kJ/Cal 10082

WEEKLY PERSONAL SUMMARY

Mood
Appetite
Energy level
Stress level
Hours of sleep **38**
Sleep quality
Injuries or illnesses: *Headache on Thursday*

kJ/Cal intake
Planned kJ/Cal **8400**
Actual kJ/Cal **10082**
Difference [+/-] **+1682**

Weight at end of week **83**
BMI at end of week **27**

EXERCISE DIARY

STRENGTH TRAINING

Exercise	Focus area	SET 1 Reps	Weight	SET 2 Reps	Weight	SET 3 Reps	Weight	SET4 Reps	Weight	Equipment	Ease
Sit ups	Stomach	10	-	10	-	10	-			Gym mat	6/10
Push ups	Arms	5	-	5	-	5	-			Gym mat	5/10
Crunches	Stomach	10	-	10	-	10	-			Gym mat	7/10

CARDIO TRAINING

Exercise	Time	Distance	Intensity	Heart rate	Ease	kJ/Cal burnt
Treadmill	20mins	4km	Hard	205	4/10	200
Treadmill	30mins	3.5km	Easy	190	7/10	120
Stepper	10mins	1.5km	Hard	200	3/10	55
Swimming	30mins	4km	Medium	198	6/10	250

Total kJ/Cal burnt **625**

INCIDENTAL EXERCISE

Day	Activity	Day	Activity
Tues	Took stairs	Sat	Played with neice
Wed	Shopping	Sun	Took the stairs
Thurs	Walk dog		
Fri	Vacuumed		
Sat	Walk dog		

MONTHLY SUMMARY

MONTH 3   **DATE** 5 / 3 / 07   **AGE** 26   **HEIGHT** 174

AVERAGE DAILY DIETARY RESULTS

Total your daily dietary results and divide by the number of days in the month to get your daily average.

Fat intake

Goal	38
Result	42
Difference [+/-]	+4

Protein intake

Goal	59
Result	57
Difference [+/-]	-2

Carbs intake

Goal	108
Result	+110
Difference [+/-]	+2

Fibre intake

Goal	25
Result	22
Difference [+/-]	-3

kJ/Cal intake

Goal	1400
Result	1520
Difference [+/-]	+120

Add up your daily results (weekly for alcohol) to get your monthly total.

Average daily coffee/teas	1
Average daily fluid intake	6
Average weekly units of alcohol	2

PHYSICAL MEASUREMENTS

LAST MTH'S GOAL		THIS MTH'S RESULT
78	Weight	80
25	BMI	26
200	Active heart rate	205
70	Resting heart rate	71
380	Recovery time	383
97	Chest	99
78	Waist	81
105	Hips	105
38	Neck	39
138	Shoulders	140
49	Right upper arm	49
49	Left upper arm	49
43	Right forearm	44
43	Left forearm	43
68	Right thigh	69
68	Left thigh	70
38	Right calf	39
38	Left calf	39

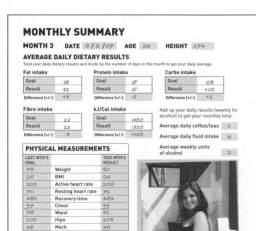

Add up your weekly planned exercise sessions to get your monthly total.

Number of planned exercise sessions this month 25

Number of completed exercise sessions this month 17

230

MONTHLY PERSONAL SUMMARY

Total your weekly results and divide by the number of weeks to get your average.

Average monthly mood	1 2 3 4 5	Average monthly appetite	1 2 3 4 5	Average monthly energy level	1 2 3 4 5
Average monthly stress level	1 2 3 4 5	Average weekly hours of sleep	40	Average monthly sleep quality	1 2 3 4 5
Average monthly stress level	1 2 3 4 5	Average weekly hours of sleep			

NEXT MONTH'S GOALS

	NEXT MTH'S GOAL		NEXT MTH'S GOAL
Fat	1150	kJ/Cal	28000
Protein	2300	Daily fluid intake	8
Carbs	6400	Daily coffee/tea intake	2
Fibre	950	Weekly alcohol intake	1

PHYSICAL MEASUREMENT GOALS

	NEXT MTH'S GOAL		NEXT MTH'S GOAL
Weight	77	Shoulders	136
BMI	25	Right upper arm	47
Active heart rate	200	Left upper arm	47
Resting heart rate	68	Right forearm	41
Recovery time	380	Left forearm	41
Chest	97	Right thigh	66
Waist	76	Left thigh	66
Hips	103	Right calf	37
Neck	36	Left calf	37

MY PERSONAL GOALS THIS MONTH

To lose 3 kg

231

YEARLY WEIGHT GRAPH

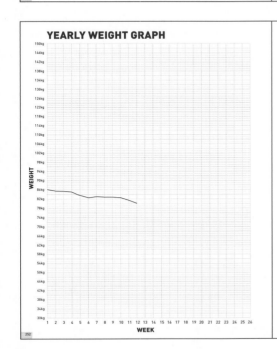

WEEK

252

Record your weekly weight and graph your progress throughout the year.

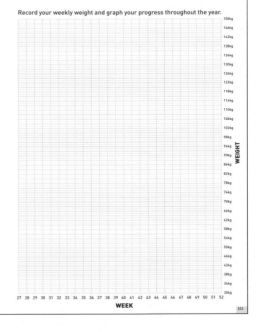

WEEK

253

TWELVE-MONTH PLANNER

	JANUARY	FEBRUARY	MARCH	APRIL	MAY	JUNE
1						
2						
3						
4						
5						
6						
7						
8						
9						
10						
11						
12						
13						
14						
15						
16						
17						
18						
19						
20						
21						
22						
23						
24						
25						
26						
27						
28						
29						
30						
31						
	JANUARY	FEBRUARY	MARCH	APRIL	MAY	JUNE

WEDNESDAY

	Time		Quantity	Fat	Protein	Carbs	Fibre	kJ/Cal
Breakfast 1 2 3 4 5 ○○○○○ HUNGER SCALE								
Mid-morning ○○○○○								
Lunch 1 2 3 4 5 ○○○○○ HUNGER SCALE								
Mid-afternoon ○○○○○								
Dinner 1 2 3 4 5 ○○○○○ HUNGER SCALE								
Evening ○○○○○								
Coffees/teas	Fluid intake ▽▽▽▽▽▽▽▽▽▽	Daily totals						

THURSDAY

	Time		Quantity	Fat	Protein	Carbs	Fibre	kJ/Cal
Breakfast 1 2 3 4 5 ○○○○○ HUNGER SCALE								
Mid-morning ○○○○○								
Lunch 1 2 3 4 5 ○○○○○ HUNGER SCALE								
Mid-afternoon ○○○○○								
Dinner 1 2 3 4 5 ○○○○○ HUNGER SCALE								
Evening ○○○○○								
Coffees/teas	Fluid intake ▽▽▽▽▽▽▽▽▽▽	Daily totals						

FRIDAY

	Time		Quantity	Fat	Protein	Carbs	Fibre	kJ/Cal
Breakfast 1 2 3 4 5 ○○○●○ HUNGER SCALE		Greek yogurt						140
Mid-morning ○○○○○								
Lunch 1 2 3 4 5 ○○○○○ HUNGER SCALE								
Mid-afternoon ○○○○○								
Dinner 1 2 3 4 5 ○○○○○ HUNGER SCALE								
Evening ○○○○○								
Coffees/teas	Fluid intake ▽▽▽▽▽▽▽▽▽▽	Daily totals						

SATURDAY

	Time		Quantity	Fat	Protein	Carbs	Fibre	kJ/Cal
Breakfast 1 2 3 4 5 ○○○○○ HUNGER SCALE								
Mid-morning ○○○○○								
Lunch 1 2 3 4 5 ○○○○○ HUNGER SCALE								
Mid-afternoon ○○○○○								
Dinner 1 2 3 4 5 ○○○○○ HUNGER SCALE								
Evening ○○○○○								

Coffees/teas [ ]   Fluid intake ⛁⛁⛁⛁⛁⛁⛁⛁⛁⛁   Daily totals

SUNDAY

	Time		Quantity	Fat	Protein	Carbs	Fibre	kJ/Cal
Breakfast 1 2 3 4 5 ○○○○○ HUNGER SCALE								
Mid-morning ○○○○○								
Lunch 1 2 3 4 5 ○○○○○ HUNGER SCALE								
Mid-afternoon ○○○○○								
Dinner 1 2 3 4 5 ○○○○○ HUNGER SCALE								
Evening ○○○○○								

Coffees/teas [ ]   Fluid intake ⛁⛁⛁⛁⛁⛁⛁⛁⛁⛁   Daily totals

Units of alcohol this week [ ]   Total alcohol kJ/Cal

Vitamins and supplements

WEEKLY TOTALS	Fat	Protein	Carbs	Fibre	kJ/Cal

WEEKLY PERSONAL SUMMARY

Mood 1 2 3 4 5 ○○○○○   **Appetite** 1 2 3 4 5 ○○○○○

Energy level 1 2 3 4 5 ○○○○○   **Stress level** 1 2 3 4 5 ○○○○○

Hours of sleep   **Sleep quality** 1 2 3 4 5 ○○○○○

Injuries or illnesses

kJ/Cal intake	
Planned kJ/Cal	
Actual kJ/Cal	
Difference [+/-]	

Weight at end of week

BMI at end of week

EXERCISE DIARY

STRENGTH TRAINING		SET 1		SET 2		SET 3		SET4			
Exercise	Focus area	Reps	Weight	Reps	Weight	Reps	Weight	Reps	Weight	Equipment	Ease

CARDIO TRAINING

Exercise	Time	Distance	Intensity	Heart rate	Ease	kJ/Cal burnt
treadmill	30 min.					

Total kJ/Cal burnt

INCIDENTAL EXERCISE

Day	Activity	Day	Activity

WEEK BEGINNING   /   /

Weight at start of week

BMI at start of week

Planned kJ/Cal this week

Possible diet-busting occasions this week

Planned exercise sessions this week

	Exercise	Completed [Y/N]
Monday		
Tuesday		
Wednesday		
Thursday		
Friday		
Saturday		
Sunday		

FOOD DIARY

MONDAY

	Time		Quantity	Fat	Protein	Carbs	Fibre	kJ/Cal
Breakfast 1 2 3 4 5 ○ ○ ○ ○ ○ HUNGER SCALE								
Mid-morning ○ ○ ○ ○ ○								
Lunch 1 2 3 4 5 ○ ○ ○ ○ ○ HUNGER SCALE								
Mid-afternoon ○ ○ ○ ○ ○								
Dinner 1 2 3 4 5 ○ ○ ○ ○ ○ HUNGER SCALE								
Evening ○ ○ ○ ○ ○								

Coffees/teas   Fluid intake ▽▽▽▽▽▽▽▽▽▽   Daily totals

TUESDAY

			Quantity	Fat	Protein	Carbs	Fibre	kJ/Cal
Breakfast 1 2 3 4 5 ○ ○ ○ ○ ○ HUNGER SCALE								
Mid-morning ○ ○ ○ ○ ○								
Lunch 1 2 3 4 5 ○ ○ ○ ○ ○ HUNGER SCALE								
Mid-afternoon ○ ○ ○ ○ ○								
Dinner 1 2 3 4 5 ○ ○ ○ ○ ○ HUNGER SCALE								
Evening ○ ○ ○ ○ ○								

Coffees/teas   Fluid intake ▽▽▽▽▽▽▽▽▽▽   Daily totals

WEDNESDAY

	Time		Quantity	Fat	Protein	Carbs	Fibre	kJ/Cal
Breakfast 1 2 3 4 5 ○○○○○ HUNGER SCALE								
Mid-morning ○○○○○								
Lunch 1 2 3 4 5 ○○○○○ HUNGER SCALE								
Mid-afternoon ○○○○○								
Dinner 1 2 3 4 5 ○○○○○ HUNGER SCALE								
Evening ○○○○○								

Coffees/teas | Fluid intake ▽▽▽▽▽▽▽▽▽▽ | Daily totals

THURSDAY

	Time		Quantity	Fat	Protein	Carbs	Fibre	kJ/Cal
Breakfast 1 2 3 4 5 ○○○○○ HUNGER SCALE								
Mid-morning ○○○○○								
Lunch 1 2 3 4 5 ○○○○○ HUNGER SCALE								
Mid-afternoon ○○○○○								
Dinner 1 2 3 4 5 ○○○○○ HUNGER SCALE								
Evening ○○○○○								

Coffees/teas | Fluid intake ▽▽▽▽▽▽▽▽▽▽ | Daily totals

FRIDAY

	Time		Quantity	Fat	Protein	Carbs	Fibre	kJ/Cal
Breakfast 1 2 3 4 5 ○○○○○ HUNGER SCALE								
Mid-morning ○○○○○								
Lunch 1 2 3 4 5 ○○○○○ HUNGER SCALE								
Mid-afternoon ○○○○○								
Dinner 1 2 3 4 5 ○○○○○ HUNGER SCALE								
Evening ○○○○○								

Coffees/teas | Fluid intake ▽▽▽▽▽▽▽▽▽▽ | Daily totals

SATURDAY

	Time		Quantity	Fat	Protein	Carbs	Fibre	kJ/Cal
Breakfast 1 2 3 4 5 ○○○○○ HUNGER SCALE								
Mid-morning ○○○○○								
Lunch 1 2 3 4 5 ○○○○○ HUNGER SCALE								
Mid-afternoon ○○○○○								
Dinner 1 2 3 4 5 ○○○○○ HUNGER SCALE								
Evening ○○○○○								

Coffees/teas ▢ Fluid intake 🥤🥤🥤🥤🥤🥤🥤🥤🥤 Daily totals

SUNDAY

	Time		Quantity	Fat	Protein	Carbs	Fibre	kJ/Cal
Breakfast 1 2 3 4 5 ○○○○○ HUNGER SCALE								
Mid-morning ○○○○○								
Lunch 1 2 3 4 5 ○○○○○ HUNGER SCALE								
Mid-afternoon ○○○○○								
Dinner 1 2 3 4 5 ○○○○○ HUNGER SCALE								
Evening ○○○○○								

Coffees/teas ▢ Fluid intake 🥤🥤🥤🥤🥤🥤🥤🥤🥤 Daily totals

Units of alcohol this week ▢ Total alcohol kJ/Cal ▢

Vitamins and supplements

WEEKLY TOTALS	Fat	Protein	Carbs	Fibre	kJ/Cal

WEEKLY PERSONAL SUMMARY

Mood 1 2 3 4 5 ○○○○○ **Appetite** 1 2 3 4 5 ○○○○○

Energy level 1 2 3 4 5 ○○○○○ **Stress level** 1 2 3 4 5 ○○○○○

Hours of sleep ▢ **Sleep quality** 1 2 3 4 5 ○○○○○

kJ/Cal intake

Planned kJ/Cal	
Actual kJ/Cal	

Difference [+/-]

Weight at end of week ▢

BMI at end of week ▢

Injuries or illnesses

EXERCISE DIARY

STRENGTH TRAINING		SET 1		SET 2		SET 3		SET4			
Exercise	Focus area	Reps	Weight	Reps	Weight	Reps	Weight	Reps	Weight	Equipment	Ease

CARDIO TRAINING

Exercise	Time	Distance	Intensity	Heart rate	Ease	kJ/Cal burnt

Total kJ/Cal burnt

INCIDENTAL EXERCISE

Day	Activity	Day	Activity

WEEK BEGINNING ___/___/___

Weight at start of week ▢

BMI at start of week ▢

Planned kJ/Cal this week ▢

Possible diet-busting occasions this week

Planned exercise sessions this week

	Exercise	Completed [Y/N]
Monday		
Tuesday		
Wednesday		
Thursday		
Friday		
Saturday		
Sunday		

FOOD DIARY

MONDAY

	Time				Quantity	Fat	Protein	Carbs	Fibre	kJ/Cal
Breakfast 1 2 3 4 5 ○○○○○ HUNGER SCALE										
Mid-morning ○○○○○										
Lunch 1 2 3 4 5 ○○○○○ HUNGER SCALE										
Mid-afternoon ○○○○○										
Dinner 1 2 3 4 5 ○○○○○ HUNGER SCALE										
Evening ○○○○○										

Coffees/teas ▢   Fluid intake ▽▽▽▽▽▽▽▽▽▽   Daily totals

TUESDAY

					Quantity	Fat	Protein	Carbs	Fibre	kJ/Cal
Breakfast 1 2 3 4 5 ○○○○○ HUNGER SCALE										
Mid-morning ○○○○○										
Lunch 1 2 3 4 5 ○○○○○ HUNGER SCALE										
Mid-afternoon ○○○○○										
Dinner 1 2 3 4 5 ○○○○○ HUNGER SCALE										
Evening ○○○○○										

Coffees/teas ▢   Fluid intake ▽▽▽▽▽▽▽▽▽▽   Daily totals

WEDNESDAY

	Time	Quantity	Fat	Protein	Carbs	Fibre	kJ/Cal
Breakfast 1 2 3 4 5 ○○○○○ HUNGER SCALE							
Mid-morning ○○○○○							
Lunch 1 2 3 4 5 ○○○○○ HUNGER SCALE							
Mid-afternoon ○○○○○							
Dinner 1 2 3 4 5 ○○○○○ HUNGER SCALE							
Evening ○○○○○							

Coffees/teas　　　Fluid intake 🥤🥤🥤🥤🥤🥤🥤🥤🥤🥤　Daily totals

THURSDAY

	Time	Quantity	Fat	Protein	Carbs	Fibre	kJ/Cal
Breakfast 1 2 3 4 5 ○○○○○ HUNGER SCALE							
Mid-morning ○○○○○							
Lunch 1 2 3 4 5 ○○○○○ HUNGER SCALE							
Mid-afternoon ○○○○○							
Dinner 1 2 3 4 5 ○○○○○ HUNGER SCALE							
Evening ○○○○○							

Coffees/teas　　　Fluid intake 🥤🥤🥤🥤🥤🥤🥤🥤🥤🥤　Daily totals

FRIDAY

	Time	Quantity	Fat	Protein	Carbs	Fibre	kJ/Cal
Breakfast 1 2 3 4 5 ○○○○○ HUNGER SCALE							
Mid-morning ○○○○○							
Lunch 1 2 3 4 5 ○○○○○ HUNGER SCALE							
Mid-afternoon ○○○○○							
Dinner 1 2 3 4 5 ○○○○○ HUNGER SCALE							
Evening ○○○○○							

Coffees/teas　　　Fluid intake 🥤🥤🥤🥤🥤🥤🥤🥤🥤🥤　Daily totals

SATURDAY

	Time		Quantity	Fat	Protein	Carbs	Fibre	kJ/Cal
Breakfast 1 2 3 4 5 ○ ○ ○ ○ ○ HUNGER SCALE								
Mid-morning ○ ○ ○ ○ ○								
Lunch 1 2 3 4 5 ○ ○ ○ ○ ○ HUNGER SCALE								
Mid-afternoon ○ ○ ○ ○ ○								
Dinner 1 2 3 4 5 ○ ○ ○ ○ ○ HUNGER SCALE								
Evening ○ ○ ○ ○ ○								

Coffees/teas ☐   Fluid intake ⊔⊔⊔⊔⊔⊔⊔⊔⊔⊔   Daily totals

SUNDAY

			Quantity	Fat	Protein	Carbs	Fibre	kJ/Cal
Breakfast 1 2 3 4 5 ○ ○ ○ ○ ○ HUNGER SCALE								
Mid-morning ○ ○ ○ ○ ○								
Lunch 1 2 3 4 5 ○ ○ ○ ○ ○ HUNGER SCALE								
Mid-afternoon ○ ○ ○ ○ ○								
Dinner 1 2 3 4 5 ○ ○ ○ ○ ○ HUNGER SCALE								
Evening ○ ○ ○ ○ ○								

Coffees/teas ☐   Fluid intake ⊔⊔⊔⊔⊔⊔⊔⊔⊔⊔   Daily totals

Units of alcohol this week ☐   **Total alcohol kJ/Cal**

Vitamins and supplements

WEEKLY TOTALS	Fat	Protein	Carbs	Fibre	kJ/Cal

WEEKLY PERSONAL SUMMARY

Mood 1 2 3 4 5 ○ ○ ○ ○ ○   **Appetite** 1 2 3 4 5 ○ ○ ○ ○ ○

Energy level 1 2 3 4 5 ○ ○ ○ ○ ○   **Stress level** 1 2 3 4 5 ○ ○ ○ ○ ○

Hours of sleep ☐   **Sleep quality** 1 2 3 4 5 ○ ○ ○ ○ ○

Injuries or illnesses

kJ/Cal intake

Planned kJ/Cal	
Actual kJ/Cal	
Difference [+/-]	

Weight at end of week

BMI at end of week

EXERCISE DIARY

STRENGTH TRAINING

Exercise	Focus area	SET 1 Reps	SET 1 Weight	SET 2 Reps	SET 2 Weight	SET 3 Reps	SET 3 Weight	SET 4 Reps	SET 4 Weight	Equipment	Ease

CARDIO TRAINING

Exercise	Time	Distance	Intensity	Heart rate	Ease	kJ/Cal burnt

Total kJ/Cal burnt

INCIDENTAL EXERCISE

Day	Activity	Day	Activity

WEEK BEGINNING   /   /

Weight at start of week

BMI at start of week

Planned kJ/Cal this week

Possible diet-busting occasions this week

Planned exercise sessions this week

	Exercise	Completed [Y/N]
Monday		
Tuesday		
Wednesday		
Thursday		
Friday		
Saturday		
Sunday		

FOOD DIARY

MONDAY

	Time					Quantity	Fat	Protein	Carbs	Fibre	kJ/Cal
Breakfast 1 2 3 4 5 ○ ○ ○ ○ ○ HUNGER SCALE											
Mid-morning ○ ○ ○ ○ ○											
Lunch 1 2 3 4 5 ○ ○ ○ ○ ○ HUNGER SCALE											
Mid-afternoon ○ ○ ○ ○ ○											
Dinner 1 2 3 4 5 ○ ○ ○ ○ ○ HUNGER SCALE											
Evening ○ ○ ○ ○ ○											

Coffees/teas   Fluid intake ☐ ☐ ☐ ☐ ☐ ☐ ☐ ☐ ☐ ☐   Daily totals

TUESDAY

	Time					Quantity	Fat	Protein	Carbs	Fibre	kJ/Cal
Breakfast 1 2 3 4 5 ○ ○ ○ ○ ○ HUNGER SCALE											
Mid-morning ○ ○ ○ ○ ○											
Lunch 1 2 3 4 5 ○ ○ ○ ○ ○ HUNGER SCALE											
Mid-afternoon ○ ○ ○ ○ ○											
Dinner 1 2 3 4 5 ○ ○ ○ ○ ○ HUNGER SCALE											
Evening ○ ○ ○ ○ ○											

Coffees/teas   Fluid intake ☐ ☐ ☐ ☐ ☐ ☐ ☐ ☐ ☐ ☐   Daily totals

WEDNESDAY

	Time		Quantity	Fat	Protein	Carbs	Fibre	kJ/Cal
Breakfast 1 2 3 4 5 ○ ○ ○ ○ ○ HUNGER SCALE								
Mid-morning ○ ○ ○ ○ ○								
Lunch 1 2 3 4 5 ○ ○ ○ ○ ○ HUNGER SCALE								
Mid-afternoon ○ ○ ○ ○ ○								
Dinner 1 2 3 4 5 ○ ○ ○ ○ ○ HUNGER SCALE								
Evening ○ ○ ○ ○ ○								

Coffees/teas ☐ Fluid intake ▽ ▽ ▽ ▽ ▽ ▽ ▽ ▽ ▽ ▽ Daily totals

THURSDAY

	Time		Quantity	Fat	Protein	Carbs	Fibre	kJ/Cal
Breakfast 1 2 3 4 5 ○ ○ ○ ○ ○ HUNGER SCALE								
Mid-morning ○ ○ ○ ○ ○								
Lunch 1 2 3 4 5 ○ ○ ○ ○ ○ HUNGER SCALE								
Mid-afternoon ○ ○ ○ ○ ○								
Dinner 1 2 3 4 5 ○ ○ ○ ○ ○ HUNGER SCALE								
Evening ○ ○ ○ ○ ○								

Coffees/teas ☐ Fluid intake ▽ ▽ ▽ ▽ ▽ ▽ ▽ ▽ ▽ ▽ Daily totals

FRIDAY

	Time		Quantity	Fat	Protein	Carbs	Fibre	kJ/Cal
Breakfast 1 2 3 4 5 ○ ○ ○ ○ ○ HUNGER SCALE								
Mid-morning ○ ○ ○ ○ ○								
Lunch 1 2 3 4 5 ○ ○ ○ ○ ○ HUNGER SCALE								
Mid-afternoon ○ ○ ○ ○ ○								
Dinner 1 2 3 4 5 ○ ○ ○ ○ ○ HUNGER SCALE								
Evening ○ ○ ○ ○ ○								

Coffees/teas ☐ Fluid intake ▽ ▽ ▽ ▽ ▽ ▽ ▽ ▽ ▽ ▽ Daily totals

SATURDAY

	Time		Quantity	Fat	Protein	Carbs	Fibre	kJ/Cal
Breakfast 1 2 3 4 5 ○○○○○ HUNGER SCALE								
Mid-morning ○○○○○								
Lunch 1 2 3 4 5 ○○○○○ HUNGER SCALE								
Mid-afternoon ○○○○○								
Dinner 1 2 3 4 5 ○○○○○ HUNGER SCALE								
Evening ○○○○○								
Coffees/teas		Fluid intake ⊔⊔⊔⊔⊔⊔⊔⊔⊔⊔	Daily totals					

SUNDAY

	Time		Quantity	Fat	Protein	Carbs	Fibre	kJ/Cal
Breakfast 1 2 3 4 5 ○○○○○ HUNGER SCALE								
Mid-morning ○○○○○								
Lunch 1 2 3 4 5 ○○○○○ HUNGER SCALE								
Mid-afternoon ○○○○○								
Dinner 1 2 3 4 5 ○○○○○ HUNGER SCALE								
Evening ○○○○○								
Coffees/teas		Fluid intake ⊔⊔⊔⊔⊔⊔⊔⊔⊔⊔	Daily totals					

Units of alcohol this week ▭   **Total alcohol kJ/Cal**

Vitamins and supplements

WEEKLY TOTALS	Fat	Protein	Carbs	Fibre	kJ/Cal

WEEKLY PERSONAL SUMMARY

Mood 1 2 3 4 5 ○○○○○   **Appetite** 1 2 3 4 5 ○○○○○

Energy level 1 2 3 4 5 ○○○○○   **Stress level** 1 2 3 4 5 ○○○○○

Hours of sleep ▭   **Sleep quality** 1 2 3 4 5 ○○○○○

kJ/Cal intake	
Planned kJ/Cal	
Actual kJ/Cal	
Difference [+/-]	

Weight at end of week

BMI at end of week

Injuries or illnesses

32

EXERCISE DIARY

STRENGTH TRAINING		SET 1		SET 2		SET 3		SET4			
Exercise	Focus area	Reps	Weight	Reps	Weight	Reps	Weight	Reps	Weight	Equipment	Ease

CARDIO TRAINING

Exercise	Time	Distance	Intensity	Heart rate	Ease	kJ/Cal burnt

Total kJ/Cal burnt

INCIDENTAL EXERCISE

Day	Activity	Day	Activity

WEEK BEGINNING   /   /

Weight at start of week

BMI at start of week

Planned kJ/Cal this week

Possible diet-busting occasions this week

Planned exercise sessions this week

	Exercise	Completed [Y/N]
Monday		
Tuesday		
Wednesday		
Thursday		
Friday		
Saturday		
Sunday		

FOOD DIARY

MONDAY

	Time		Quantity	Fat	Protein	Carbs	Fibre	kJ/Cal
Breakfast 1 2 3 4 5 ○○○○○ HUNGER SCALE								
Mid-morning ○○○○○								
Lunch 1 2 3 4 5 ○○○○○ HUNGER SCALE								
Mid-afternoon ○○○○○								
Dinner 1 2 3 4 5 ○○○○○ HUNGER SCALE								
Evening ○○○○○								

Coffees/teas   Fluid intake ☐☐☐☐☐☐☐☐☐☐   Daily totals

TUESDAY

	Time		Quantity	Fat	Protein	Carbs	Fibre	kJ/Cal
Breakfast 1 2 3 4 5 ○○○○○ HUNGER SCALE								
Mid-morning ○○○○○								
Lunch 1 2 3 4 5 ○○○○○ HUNGER SCALE								
Mid-afternoon ○○○○○								
Dinner 1 2 3 4 5 ○○○○○ HUNGER SCALE								
Evening ○○○○○								

Coffees/teas   Fluid intake ☐☐☐☐☐☐☐☐☐☐   Daily totals

WEDNESDAY

	Time		Quantity	Fat	Protein	Carbs	Fibre	kJ/Cal
Breakfast 1 2 3 4 5 ○ ○ ○ ○ ○ HUNGER SCALE								
Mid-morning ○ ○ ○ ○ ○								
Lunch 1 2 3 4 5 ○ ○ ○ ○ ○ HUNGER SCALE								
Mid-afternoon ○ ○ ○ ○ ○								
Dinner 1 2 3 4 5 ○ ○ ○ ○ ○ HUNGER SCALE								
Evening ○ ○ ○ ○ ○								
Coffees/teas		Fluid intake ☐☐☐☐☐☐☐☐☐☐	Daily totals					

THURSDAY

	Time		Quantity	Fat	Protein	Carbs	Fibre	kJ/Cal
Breakfast 1 2 3 4 5 ○ ○ ○ ○ ○ HUNGER SCALE								
Mid-morning ○ ○ ○ ○ ○								
Lunch 1 2 3 4 5 ○ ○ ○ ○ ○ HUNGER SCALE								
Mid-afternoon ○ ○ ○ ○ ○								
Dinner 1 2 3 4 5 ○ ○ ○ ○ ○ HUNGER SCALE								
Evening ○ ○ ○ ○ ○								
Coffees/teas		Fluid intake ☐☐☐☐☐☐☐☐☐☐	Daily totals					

FRIDAY

	Time		Quantity	Fat	Protein	Carbs	Fibre	kJ/Cal
Breakfast 1 2 3 4 5 ○ ○ ○ ○ ○ HUNGER SCALE								
Mid-morning ○ ○ ○ ○ ○								
Lunch 1 2 3 4 5 ○ ○ ○ ○ ○ HUNGER SCALE								
Mid-afternoon ○ ○ ○ ○ ○								
Dinner 1 2 3 4 5 ○ ○ ○ ○ ○ HUNGER SCALE								
Evening ○ ○ ○ ○ ○								
Coffees/teas		Fluid intake ☐☐☐☐☐☐☐☐☐☐	Daily totals					

SATURDAY

	Time		Quantity	Fat	Protein	Carbs	Fibre	kJ/Cal
Breakfast 1 2 3 4 5 ○ ○ ○ ○ ○ HUNGER SCALE								
Mid-morning ○ ○ ○ ○ ○								
Lunch 1 2 3 4 5 ○ ○ ○ ○ ○ HUNGER SCALE								
Mid-afternoon ○ ○ ○ ○ ○								
Dinner 1 2 3 4 5 ○ ○ ○ ○ ○ HUNGER SCALE								
Evening ○ ○ ○ ○ ○								

Coffees/teas ▢ Fluid intake ⊔⊔⊔⊔⊔⊔⊔⊔⊔⊔ Daily totals

SUNDAY

	Time		Quantity	Fat	Protein	Carbs	Fibre	kJ/Cal
Breakfast 1 2 3 4 5 ○ ○ ○ ○ ○ HUNGER SCALE								
Mid-morning ○ ○ ○ ○ ○								
Lunch 1 2 3 4 5 ○ ○ ○ ○ ○ HUNGER SCALE								
Mid-afternoon ○ ○ ○ ○ ○								
Dinner 1 2 3 4 5 ○ ○ ○ ○ ○ HUNGER SCALE								
Evening ○ ○ ○ ○ ○								

Coffees/teas ▢ Fluid intake ⊔⊔⊔⊔⊔⊔⊔⊔⊔⊔ Daily totals

Units of alcohol this week ▢   Total alcohol kJ/Cal ▢

Vitamins and supplements

	Fat	Protein	Carbs	Fibre	kJ/Cal
WEEKLY TOTALS					

WEEKLY PERSONAL SUMMARY

Mood 1 2 3 4 5 ○ ○ ○ ○ ○   **Appetite** 1 2 3 4 5 ○ ○ ○ ○ ○

Energy level 1 2 3 4 5 ○ ○ ○ ○ ○   **Stress level** 1 2 3 4 5 ○ ○ ○ ○ ○

Hours of sleep ▢   **Sleep quality** 1 2 3 4 5 ○ ○ ○ ○ ○

Injuries or illnesses

kJ/Cal intake

Planned kJ/Cal	
Actual kJ/Cal	

Difference [+/-]

Weight at end of week

BMI at end of week

EXERCISE DIARY

STRENGTH TRAINING		SET 1		SET 2		SET 3		SET4			
Exercise	Focus area	Reps	Weight	Reps	Weight	Reps	Weight	Reps	Weight	Equipment	Ease

CARDIO TRAINING

Exercise	Time	Distance	Intensity	Heart rate	Ease	kJ/Cal burnt

Total kJ/Cal burnt

INCIDENTAL EXERCISE

Day	Activity	Day	Activity

WEEK BEGINNING ___ / ___ / ___

Weight at start of week _____

BMI at start of week _____

Planned kJ/Cal this week _____

Possible diet-busting occasions this week

Planned exercise sessions this week

	Exercise	Completed [Y/N]
Monday		
Tuesday		
Wednesday		
Thursday		
Friday		
Saturday		
Sunday		

FOOD DIARY

MONDAY

	Time		Quantity	Fat	Protein	Carbs	Fibre	kJ/Cal
Breakfast 1 2 3 4 5 ○○○○○ HUNGER SCALE								
Mid-morning ○○○○○								
Lunch 1 2 3 4 5 ○○○○○ HUNGER SCALE								
Mid-afternoon ○○○○○								
Dinner 1 2 3 4 5 ○○○○○ HUNGER SCALE								
Evening ○○○○○								

Coffees/teas _____ Fluid intake ▽▽▽▽▽▽▽▽▽▽ Daily totals

TUESDAY

	Time		Quantity	Fat	Protein	Carbs	Fibre	kJ/Cal
Breakfast 1 2 3 4 5 ○○○○○ HUNGER SCALE								
Mid-morning ○○○○○								
Lunch 1 2 3 4 5 ○○○○○ HUNGER SCALE								
Mid-afternoon ○○○○○								
Dinner 1 2 3 4 5 ○○○○○ HUNGER SCALE								
Evening ○○○○○								

Coffees/teas _____ Fluid intake ▽▽▽▽▽▽▽▽▽▽ Daily totals

WEDNESDAY	Time		Quantity	Fat	Protein	Carbs	Fibre	kJ/Cal
Breakfast 1 2 3 4 5 ○ ○ ○ ○ ○ HUNGER SCALE								
Mid-morning ○ ○ ○ ○ ○								
Lunch 1 2 3 4 5 ○ ○ ○ ○ ○ HUNGER SCALE								
Mid-afternoon ○ ○ ○ ○ ○								
Dinner 1 2 3 4 5 ○ ○ ○ ○ ○ HUNGER SCALE								
Evening ○ ○ ○ ○ ○								

Coffees/teas   Fluid intake ☐☐☐☐☐☐☐☐☐☐   Daily totals

THURSDAY								
Breakfast 1 2 3 4 5 ○ ○ ○ ○ ○ HUNGER SCALE								
Mid-morning ○ ○ ○ ○ ○								
Lunch 1 2 3 4 5 ○ ○ ○ ○ ○ HUNGER SCALE								
Mid-afternoon ○ ○ ○ ○ ○								
Dinner 1 2 3 4 5 ○ ○ ○ ○ ○ HUNGER SCALE								
Evening ○ ○ ○ ○ ○								

Coffees/teas   Fluid intake ☐☐☐☐☐☐☐☐☐☐   Daily totals

FRIDAY								
Breakfast 1 2 3 4 5 ○ ○ ○ ○ ○ HUNGER SCALE								
Mid-morning ○ ○ ○ ○ ○								
Lunch 1 2 3 4 5 ○ ○ ○ ○ ○ HUNGER SCALE								
Mid-afternoon ○ ○ ○ ○ ○								
Dinner 1 2 3 4 5 ○ ○ ○ ○ ○ HUNGER SCALE								
Evening ○ ○ ○ ○ ○								

Coffees/teas   Fluid intake ☐☐☐☐☐☐☐☐☐☐   Daily totals

SATURDAY

	Time		Quantity	Fat	Protein	Carbs	Fibre	kJ/Cal
Breakfast 1 2 3 4 5 ○○○○○ HUNGER SCALE								
Mid-morning ○○○○○								
Lunch 1 2 3 4 5 ○○○○○ HUNGER SCALE								
Mid-afternoon ○○○○○								
Dinner 1 2 3 4 5 ○○○○○ HUNGER SCALE								
Evening ○○○○○								

Coffees/teas ____   Fluid intake 🥤🥤🥤🥤🥤🥤🥤🥤🥤🥤   Daily totals ____

SUNDAY

	Time		Quantity	Fat	Protein	Carbs	Fibre	kJ/Cal
Breakfast 1 2 3 4 5 ○○○○○ HUNGER SCALE								
Mid-morning ○○○○○								
Lunch 1 2 3 4 5 ○○○○○ HUNGER SCALE								
Mid-afternoon ○○○○○								
Dinner 1 2 3 4 5 ○○○○○ HUNGER SCALE								
Evening ○○○○○								

Coffees/teas ____   Fluid intake 🥤🥤🥤🥤🥤🥤🥤🥤🥤🥤   Daily totals ____

Units of alcohol this week ____   Total alcohol kJ/Cal ____

Vitamins and supplements ____

WEEKLY TOTALS	Fat	Protein	Carbs	Fibre	kJ/Cal

WEEKLY PERSONAL SUMMARY

Mood 1 2 3 4 5 ○○○○○   **Appetite** 1 2 3 4 5 ○○○○○

Energy level 1 2 3 4 5 ○○○○○   **Stress level** 1 2 3 4 5 ○○○○○

Hours of sleep ____   **Sleep quality** 1 2 3 4 5 ○○○○○

kJ/Cal intake

Planned kJ/Cal	
Actual kJ/Cal	

Difference [+/-]

Weight at end of week ____

BMI at end of week ____

Injuries or illnesses ____

40

EXERCISE DIARY

STRENGTH TRAINING		SET 1		SET 2		SET 3		SET4			
Exercise	Focus area	Reps	Weight	Reps	Weight	Reps	Weight	Reps	Weight	Equipment	Ease

CARDIO TRAINING

Exercise	Time	Distance	Intensity	Heart rate	Ease	kJ/Cal burnt

Total kJ/Cal burnt

INCIDENTAL EXERCISE

Day	Activity	Day	Activity

WEEK BEGINNING ___ / ___ / ___

Weight at start of week ▢

BMI at start of week ▢

Planned kJ/Cal this week ▢

Possible diet-busting occasions this week

▢

Planned exercise sessions this week

	Exercise	Completed [Y/N]
Monday		
Tuesday		
Wednesday		
Thursday		
Friday		
Saturday		
Sunday		

FOOD DIARY

MONDAY

	Time		Quantity	Fat	Protein	Carbs	Fibre	kJ/Cal
Breakfast 1 2 3 4 5 ○ ○ ○ ○ ○ HUNGER SCALE								
Mid-morning ○ ○ ○ ○ ○								
Lunch 1 2 3 4 5 ○ ○ ○ ○ ○ HUNGER SCALE								
Mid-afternoon ○ ○ ○ ○ ○								
Dinner 1 2 3 4 5 ○ ○ ○ ○ ○ HUNGER SCALE								
Evening ○ ○ ○ ○ ○								

Coffees/teas ▢   Fluid intake ▭▭▭▭▭▭▭▭▭▭   Daily totals

TUESDAY

	Time		Quantity	Fat	Protein	Carbs	Fibre	kJ/Cal
Breakfast 1 2 3 4 5 ○ ○ ○ ○ ○ HUNGER SCALE								
Mid-morning ○ ○ ○ ○ ○								
Lunch 1 2 3 4 5 ○ ○ ○ ○ ○ HUNGER SCALE								
Mid-afternoon ○ ○ ○ ○ ○								
Dinner 1 2 3 4 5 ○ ○ ○ ○ ○ HUNGER SCALE								
Evening ○ ○ ○ ○ ○								

Coffees/teas ▢   Fluid intake ▭▭▭▭▭▭▭▭▭▭   Daily totals

WEDNESDAY

	Time		Quantity	Fat	Protein	Carbs	Fibre	kJ/Cal
Breakfast 1 2 3 4 5 ○ ○ ○ ○ ○ HUNGER SCALE								
Mid-morning ○ ○ ○ ○ ○								
Lunch 1 2 3 4 5 ○ ○ ○ ○ ○ HUNGER SCALE								
Mid-afternoon ○ ○ ○ ○ ○								
Dinner 1 2 3 4 5 ○ ○ ○ ○ ○ HUNGER SCALE								
Evening ○ ○ ○ ○ ○								

Coffees/teas ▢   Fluid intake ▽▽▽▽▽▽▽▽▽▽   Daily totals

THURSDAY

	Time		Quantity	Fat	Protein	Carbs	Fibre	kJ/Cal
Breakfast 1 2 3 4 5 ○ ○ ○ ○ ○ HUNGER SCALE								
Mid-morning ○ ○ ○ ○ ○								
Lunch 1 2 3 4 5 ○ ○ ○ ○ ○ HUNGER SCALE								
Mid-afternoon ○ ○ ○ ○ ○								
Dinner 1 2 3 4 5 ○ ○ ○ ○ ○ HUNGER SCALE								
Evening ○ ○ ○ ○ ○								

Coffees/teas ▢   Fluid intake ▽▽▽▽▽▽▽▽▽▽   Daily totals

FRIDAY

	Time		Quantity	Fat	Protein	Carbs	Fibre	kJ/Cal
Breakfast 1 2 3 4 5 ○ ○ ○ ○ ○ HUNGER SCALE								
Mid-morning ○ ○ ○ ○ ○								
Lunch 1 2 3 4 5 ○ ○ ○ ○ ○ HUNGER SCALE								
Mid-afternoon ○ ○ ○ ○ ○								
Dinner 1 2 3 4 5 ○ ○ ○ ○ ○ HUNGER SCALE								
Evening ○ ○ ○ ○ ○								

Coffees/teas ▢   Fluid intake ▽▽▽▽▽▽▽▽▽▽   Daily totals

SATURDAY

	Time		Quantity	Fat	Protein	Carbs	Fibre	kJ/Cal
Breakfast 1 2 3 4 5 ○○○○○ HUNGER SCALE								
Mid-morning ○○○○○								
Lunch 1 2 3 4 5 ○○○○○ HUNGER SCALE								
Mid-afternoon ○○○○○								
Dinner 1 2 3 4 5 ○○○○○ HUNGER SCALE								
Evening ○○○○○								

Coffees/teas   Fluid intake ▽▽▽▽▽▽▽▽▽▽   Daily totals

SUNDAY

	Time		Quantity	Fat	Protein	Carbs	Fibre	kJ/Cal
Breakfast 1 2 3 4 5 ○○○○○ HUNGER SCALE								
Mid-morning ○○○○○								
Lunch 1 2 3 4 5 ○○○○○ HUNGER SCALE								
Mid-afternoon ○○○○○								
Dinner 1 2 3 4 5 ○○○○○ HUNGER SCALE								
Evening ○○○○○								

Coffees/teas   Fluid intake ▽▽▽▽▽▽▽▽▽▽   Daily totals

Units of alcohol this week   **Total alcohol kJ/Cal**

Vitamins and supplements

	Fat	Protein	Carbs	Fibre	kJ/Cal
WEEKLY TOTALS					

WEEKLY PERSONAL SUMMARY

Mood 1 2 3 4 5 ○○○○○   **Appetite** 1 2 3 4 5 ○○○○○

Energy level 1 2 3 4 5 ○○○○○   **Stress level** 1 2 3 4 5 ○○○○○

Hours of sleep   **Sleep quality** 1 2 3 4 5 ○○○○○

Injuries or illnesses

kJ/Cal intake

Planned kJ/Cal	
Actual kJ/Cal	
Difference [+/-]	

Weight at end of week

BMI at end of week

EXERCISE DIARY

STRENGTH TRAINING		SET 1		SET 2		SET 3		SET4			
Exercise	Focus area	Reps	Weight	Reps	Weight	Reps	Weight	Reps	Weight	Equipment	Ease

CARDIO TRAINING

Exercise	Time	Distance	Intensity	Heart rate	Ease	kJ/Cal burnt

Total kJ/Cal burnt

INCIDENTAL EXERCISE

Day	Activity	Day	Activity

WEEK BEGINNING   /   /

Weight at start of week

BMI at start of week

Planned kJ/Cal this week

Possible diet-busting occasions this week

Planned exercise sessions this week

	Exercise	Completed [Y/N]
Monday		
Tuesday		
Wednesday		
Thursday		
Friday		
Saturday		
Sunday		

FOOD DIARY

MONDAY

	Time		Quantity	Fat	Protein	Carbs	Fibre	kJ/Cal
Breakfast 1 2 3 4 5 ○ ○ ○ ○ ○ HUNGER SCALE								
Mid-morning ○ ○ ○ ○ ○								
Lunch 1 2 3 4 5 ○ ○ ○ ○ ○ HUNGER SCALE								
Mid-afternoon ○ ○ ○ ○ ○								
Dinner 1 2 3 4 5 ○ ○ ○ ○ ○ HUNGER SCALE								
Evening ○ ○ ○ ○ ○								

Coffees/teas   Fluid intake ⛾⛾⛾⛾⛾⛾⛾⛾⛾⛾   Daily totals

TUESDAY

	Time		Quantity	Fat	Protein	Carbs	Fibre	kJ/Cal
Breakfast 1 2 3 4 5 ○ ○ ○ ○ ○ HUNGER SCALE								
Mid-morning ○ ○ ○ ○ ○								
Lunch 1 2 3 4 5 ○ ○ ○ ○ ○ HUNGER SCALE								
Mid-afternoon ○ ○ ○ ○ ○								
Dinner 1 2 3 4 5 ○ ○ ○ ○ ○ HUNGER SCALE								
Evening ○ ○ ○ ○ ○								

Coffees/teas   Fluid intake ⛾⛾⛾⛾⛾⛾⛾⛾⛾⛾   Daily totals

WEDNESDAY

	Time		Quantity	Fat	Protein	Carbs	Fibre	kJ/Cal
Breakfast 1 2 3 4 5 ○○○○○ HUNGER SCALE								
Mid-morning ○○○○○								
Lunch 1 2 3 4 5 ○○○○○ HUNGER SCALE								
Mid-afternoon ○○○○○								
Dinner 1 2 3 4 5 ○○○○○ HUNGER SCALE								
Evening ○○○○○								

Coffees/teas [ ]   Fluid intake ▽▽▽▽▽▽▽▽▽▽   Daily totals

THURSDAY

Breakfast 1 2 3 4 5 ○○○○○ HUNGER SCALE								
Mid-morning ○○○○○								
Lunch 1 2 3 4 5 ○○○○○ HUNGER SCALE								
Mid-afternoon ○○○○○								
Dinner 1 2 3 4 5 ○○○○○ HUNGER SCALE								
Evening ○○○○○								

Coffees/teas [ ]   Fluid intake ▽▽▽▽▽▽▽▽▽▽   Daily totals

FRIDAY

Breakfast 1 2 3 4 5 ○○○○○ HUNGER SCALE								
Mid-morning ○○○○○								
Lunch 1 2 3 4 5 ○○○○○ HUNGER SCALE								
Mid-afternoon ○○○○○								
Dinner 1 2 3 4 5 ○○○○○ HUNGER SCALE								
Evening ○○○○○								

Coffees/teas [ ]   Fluid intake ▽▽▽▽▽▽▽▽▽▽   Daily totals

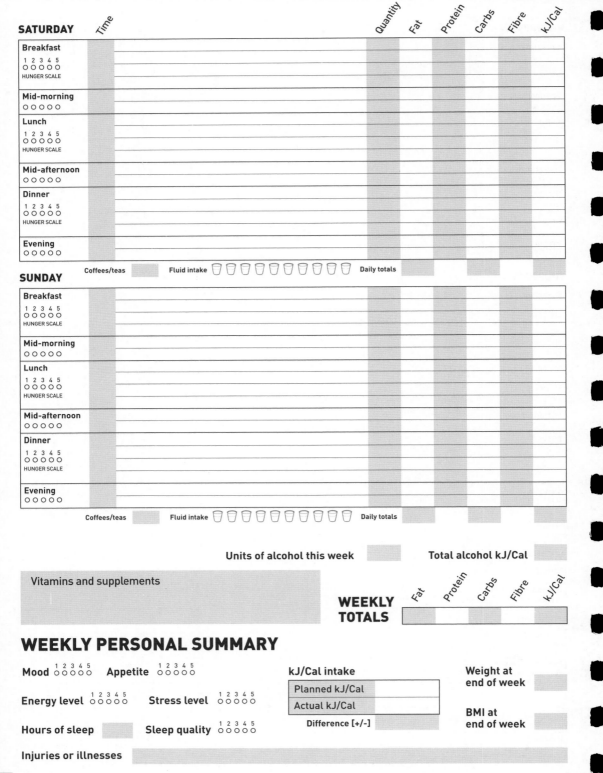

SATURDAY

	Time			Quantity	Fat	Protein	Carbs	Fibre	kJ/Cal
Breakfast 1 2 3 4 5 ○○○○○ HUNGER SCALE									
Mid-morning ○○○○○									
Lunch 1 2 3 4 5 ○○○○○ HUNGER SCALE									
Mid-afternoon ○○○○○									
Dinner 1 2 3 4 5 ○○○○○ HUNGER SCALE									
Evening ○○○○○									

Coffees/teas   Fluid intake ▭▭▭▭▭▭▭▭▭▭   Daily totals

SUNDAY

	Time			Quantity	Fat	Protein	Carbs	Fibre	kJ/Cal
Breakfast 1 2 3 4 5 ○○○○○ HUNGER SCALE									
Mid-morning ○○○○○									
Lunch 1 2 3 4 5 ○○○○○ HUNGER SCALE									
Mid-afternoon ○○○○○									
Dinner 1 2 3 4 5 ○○○○○ HUNGER SCALE									
Evening ○○○○○									

Coffees/teas   Fluid intake ▭▭▭▭▭▭▭▭▭▭   Daily totals

Units of alcohol this week   Total alcohol kJ/Cal

Vitamins and supplements

WEEKLY TOTALS	Fat	Protein	Carbs	Fibre	kJ/Cal

WEEKLY PERSONAL SUMMARY

Mood 1 2 3 4 5 ○○○○○   **Appetite** 1 2 3 4 5 ○○○○○

Energy level 1 2 3 4 5 ○○○○○   **Stress level** 1 2 3 4 5 ○○○○○

Hours of sleep   **Sleep quality** 1 2 3 4 5 ○○○○○

Injuries or illnesses

kJ/Cal intake

Planned kJ/Cal	
Actual kJ/Cal	
Difference [+/-]	

Weight at end of week

BMI at end of week

EXERCISE DIARY

STRENGTH TRAINING

Exercise	Focus area	SET 1		SET 2		SET 3		SET4		Equipment	Ease
		Reps	Weight	Reps	Weight	Reps	Weight	Reps	Weight		

CARDIO TRAINING

Exercise	Time	Distance	Intensity	Heart rate	Ease	kJ/Cal burnt

Total kJ/Cal burnt

INCIDENTAL EXERCISE

Day	Activity	Day	Activity

WEEK BEGINNING / /

Weight at start of week

BMI at start of week

Planned kJ/Cal this week

Possible diet-busting occasions this week

Planned exercise sessions this week

	Exercise	Completed [Y/N]
Monday		
Tuesday		
Wednesday		
Thursday		
Friday		
Saturday		
Sunday		

FOOD DIARY

MONDAY

	Time		Quantity	Fat	Protein	Carbs	Fibre	kJ/Cal
Breakfast 1 2 3 4 5 ○○○○○ HUNGER SCALE								
Mid-morning ○○○○○								
Lunch 1 2 3 4 5 ○○○○○ HUNGER SCALE								
Mid-afternoon ○○○○○								
Dinner 1 2 3 4 5 ○○○○○ HUNGER SCALE								
Evening ○○○○○								

Coffees/teas   Fluid intake ☐☐☐☐☐☐☐☐☐☐   Daily totals

TUESDAY

	Time		Quantity	Fat	Protein	Carbs	Fibre	kJ/Cal
Breakfast 1 2 3 4 5 ○○○○○ HUNGER SCALE								
Mid-morning ○○○○○								
Lunch 1 2 3 4 5 ○○○○○ HUNGER SCALE								
Mid-afternoon ○○○○○								
Dinner 1 2 3 4 5 ○○○○○ HUNGER SCALE								
Evening ○○○○○								

Coffees/teas   Fluid intake ☐☐☐☐☐☐☐☐☐☐   Daily totals

	Time							Quantity	Fat	Protein	Carbs	Fibre	kJ/Cal

WEDNESDAY

Breakfast
1 2 3 4 5
○ ○ ○ ○ ○
HUNGER SCALE

Mid-morning
○ ○ ○ ○ ○

Lunch
1 2 3 4 5
○ ○ ○ ○ ○
HUNGER SCALE

Mid-afternoon
○ ○ ○ ○ ○

Dinner
1 2 3 4 5
○ ○ ○ ○ ○
HUNGER SCALE

Evening
○ ○ ○ ○ ○

Coffees/teas   Fluid intake ▽▽▽▽▽▽▽▽▽▽   Daily totals

THURSDAY

Breakfast
1 2 3 4 5
○ ○ ○ ○ ○
HUNGER SCALE

Mid-morning
○ ○ ○ ○ ○

Lunch
1 2 3 4 5
○ ○ ○ ○ ○
HUNGER SCALE

Mid-afternoon
○ ○ ○ ○ ○

Dinner
1 2 3 4 5
○ ○ ○ ○ ○
HUNGER SCALE

Evening
○ ○ ○ ○ ○

Coffees/teas   Fluid intake ▽▽▽▽▽▽▽▽▽▽   Daily totals

FRIDAY

Breakfast
1 2 3 4 5
○ ○ ○ ○ ○
HUNGER SCALE

Mid-morning
○ ○ ○ ○ ○

Lunch
1 2 3 4 5
○ ○ ○ ○ ○
HUNGER SCALE

Mid-afternoon
○ ○ ○ ○ ○

Dinner
1 2 3 4 5
○ ○ ○ ○ ○
HUNGER SCALE

Evening
○ ○ ○ ○ ○

Coffees/teas   Fluid intake ▽▽▽▽▽▽▽▽▽▽   Daily totals

SATURDAY

	Time		Quantity	Fat	Protein	Carbs	Fibre	kJ/Cal
Breakfast 1 2 3 4 5 ○ ○ ○ ○ ○ HUNGER SCALE								
Mid-morning ○ ○ ○ ○ ○								
Lunch 1 2 3 4 5 ○ ○ ○ ○ ○ HUNGER SCALE								
Mid-afternoon ○ ○ ○ ○ ○								
Dinner 1 2 3 4 5 ○ ○ ○ ○ ○ HUNGER SCALE								
Evening ○ ○ ○ ○ ○								

Coffees/teas ▢ Fluid intake ▽▽▽▽▽▽▽▽▽▽ Daily totals

SUNDAY

	Time		Quantity	Fat	Protein	Carbs	Fibre	kJ/Cal
Breakfast 1 2 3 4 5 ○ ○ ○ ○ ○ HUNGER SCALE								
Mid-morning ○ ○ ○ ○ ○								
Lunch 1 2 3 4 5 ○ ○ ○ ○ ○ HUNGER SCALE								
Mid-afternoon ○ ○ ○ ○ ○								
Dinner 1 2 3 4 5 ○ ○ ○ ○ ○ HUNGER SCALE								
Evening ○ ○ ○ ○ ○								

Coffees/teas ▢ Fluid intake ▽▽▽▽▽▽▽▽▽▽ Daily totals

Units of alcohol this week ▢   Total alcohol kJ/Cal ▢

Vitamins and supplements

WEEKLY TOTALS	Fat	Protein	Carbs	Fibre	kJ/Cal

WEEKLY PERSONAL SUMMARY

Mood 1 2 3 4 5 ○ ○ ○ ○ ○   **Appetite** 1 2 3 4 5 ○ ○ ○ ○ ○

Energy level 1 2 3 4 5 ○ ○ ○ ○ ○   **Stress level** 1 2 3 4 5 ○ ○ ○ ○ ○

Hours of sleep ▢   **Sleep quality** 1 2 3 4 5 ○ ○ ○ ○ ○

Injuries or illnesses

kJ/Cal intake

Planned kJ/Cal	
Actual kJ/Cal	

Difference [+/-]

Weight at end of week

BMI at end of week

EXERCISE DIARY

STRENGTH TRAINING		SET 1		SET 2		SET 3		SET4			
Exercise	Focus area	Reps	Weight	Reps	Weight	Reps	Weight	Reps	Weight	Equipment	Ease

CARDIO TRAINING

Exercise	Time	Distance	Intensity	Heart rate	Ease	kJ/Cal burnt

Total kJ/Cal burnt

INCIDENTAL EXERCISE

Day	Activity	Day	Activity

WEEK BEGINNING / /

Weight at start of week ☐

BMI at start of week ☐

Planned kJ/Cal this week ☐

Possible diet-busting occasions this week

Planned exercise sessions this week

	Exercise	Completed [Y/N]
Monday		
Tuesday		
Wednesday		
Thursday		
Friday		
Saturday		
Sunday		

FOOD DIARY

MONDAY

	Time		Quantity	Fat	Protein	Carbs	Fibre	kJ/Cal
Breakfast 1 2 3 4 5 ○○○○ HUNGER SCALE								
Mid-morning ○○○○○								
Lunch 1 2 3 4 5 ○○○○ HUNGER SCALE								
Mid-afternoon ○○○○○								
Dinner 1 2 3 4 5 ○○○○ HUNGER SCALE								
Evening ○○○○○								

Coffees/teas ☐   Fluid intake ☐☐☐☐☐☐☐☐☐☐   Daily totals

TUESDAY

	Time		Quantity	Fat	Protein	Carbs	Fibre	kJ/Cal
Breakfast 1 2 3 4 5 ○○○○ HUNGER SCALE								
Mid-morning ○○○○○								
Lunch 1 2 3 4 5 ○○○○ HUNGER SCALE								
Mid-afternoon ○○○○○								
Dinner 1 2 3 4 5 ○○○○ HUNGER SCALE								
Evening ○○○○○								

Coffees/teas ☐   Fluid intake ☐☐☐☐☐☐☐☐☐☐   Daily totals

WEDNESDAY

	Time		Quantity	Fat	Protein	Carbs	Fibre	kJ/Cal
Breakfast 1 2 3 4 5 ○○○○○ HUNGER SCALE								
Mid-morning ○○○○○								
Lunch 1 2 3 4 5 ○○○○○ HUNGER SCALE								
Mid-afternoon ○○○○○								
Dinner 1 2 3 4 5 ○○○○○ HUNGER SCALE								
Evening ○○○○○								

Coffees/teas [ ] Fluid intake ▽▽▽▽▽▽▽▽▽▽ Daily totals

THURSDAY

	Time		Quantity	Fat	Protein	Carbs	Fibre	kJ/Cal
Breakfast 1 2 3 4 5 ○○○○○ HUNGER SCALE								
Mid-morning ○○○○○								
Lunch 1 2 3 4 5 ○○○○○ HUNGER SCALE								
Mid-afternoon ○○○○○								
Dinner 1 2 3 4 5 ○○○○○ HUNGER SCALE								
Evening ○○○○○								

Coffees/teas [ ] Fluid intake ▽▽▽▽▽▽▽▽▽▽ Daily totals

FRIDAY

	Time		Quantity	Fat	Protein	Carbs	Fibre	kJ/Cal
Breakfast 1 2 3 4 5 ○○○○○ HUNGER SCALE								
Mid-morning ○○○○○								
Lunch 1 2 3 4 5 ○○○○○ HUNGER SCALE								
Mid-afternoon ○○○○○								
Dinner 1 2 3 4 5 ○○○○○ HUNGER SCALE								
Evening ○○○○○								

Coffees/teas [ ] Fluid intake ▽▽▽▽▽▽▽▽▽▽ Daily totals

SATURDAY

	Time		Quantity	Fat	Protein	Carbs	Fibre	kJ/Cal
Breakfast 1 2 3 4 5 ○○○○○ HUNGER SCALE								
Mid-morning ○○○○○								
Lunch 1 2 3 4 5 ○○○○○ HUNGER SCALE								
Mid-afternoon ○○○○○								
Dinner 1 2 3 4 5 ○○○○○ HUNGER SCALE								
Evening ○○○○○								

Coffees/teas   Fluid intake ▽▽▽▽▽▽▽▽▽▽   Daily totals

SUNDAY

	Time		Quantity	Fat	Protein	Carbs	Fibre	kJ/Cal
Breakfast 1 2 3 4 5 ○○○○○ HUNGER SCALE								
Mid-morning ○○○○○								
Lunch 1 2 3 4 5 ○○○○○ HUNGER SCALE								
Mid-afternoon ○○○○○								
Dinner 1 2 3 4 5 ○○○○○ HUNGER SCALE								
Evening ○○○○○								

Coffees/teas   Fluid intake ▽▽▽▽▽▽▽▽▽▽   Daily totals

Units of alcohol this week   **Total alcohol kJ/Cal**

Vitamins and supplements

WEEKLY TOTALS	Fat	Protein	Carbs	Fibre	kJ/Cal

WEEKLY PERSONAL SUMMARY

Mood 1 2 3 4 5 ○○○○○   **Appetite** 1 2 3 4 5 ○○○○○

Energy level 1 2 3 4 5 ○○○○○   **Stress level** 1 2 3 4 5 ○○○○○

Hours of sleep   **Sleep quality** 1 2 3 4 5 ○○○○○

Injuries or illnesses

kJ/Cal intake	
Planned kJ/Cal	
Actual kJ/Cal	
Difference [+/-]	

Weight at end of week

BMI at end of week

EXERCISE DIARY

STRENGTH TRAINING		SET 1		SET 2		SET 3		SET4			
Exercise	Focus area	Reps	Weight	Reps	Weight	Reps	Weight	Reps	Weight	Equipment	Ease

CARDIO TRAINING

Exercise	Time	Distance	Intensity	Heart rate	Ease	kJ/Cal burnt

Total kJ/Cal burnt

INCIDENTAL EXERCISE

Day	Activity	Day	Activity

WEEK BEGINNING   /   /

Weight at start of week

BMI at start of week

Planned kJ/Cal this week

Possible diet-busting occasions this week

Planned exercise sessions this week

	Exercise	Completed [Y/N]
Monday		
Tuesday		
Wednesday		
Thursday		
Friday		
Saturday		
Sunday		

FOOD DIARY

MONDAY

	Time		Quantity	Fat	Protein	Carbs	Fibre	kJ/Cal
Breakfast 1 2 3 4 5 ○○○○○ HUNGER SCALE								
Mid-morning ○○○○○								
Lunch 1 2 3 4 5 ○○○○○ HUNGER SCALE								
Mid-afternoon ○○○○○								
Dinner 1 2 3 4 5 ○○○○○ HUNGER SCALE								
Evening ○○○○○								

Coffees/teas   Fluid intake ▽▽▽▽▽▽▽▽▽▽   Daily totals

TUESDAY

Breakfast 1 2 3 4 5 ○○○○○ HUNGER SCALE								
Mid-morning ○○○○○								
Lunch 1 2 3 4 5 ○○○○○ HUNGER SCALE								
Mid-afternoon ○○○○○								
Dinner 1 2 3 4 5 ○○○○○ HUNGER SCALE								
Evening ○○○○○								

Coffees/teas   Fluid intake ▽▽▽▽▽▽▽▽▽▽   Daily totals

WEDNESDAY

	Time		Quantity	Fat	Protein	Carbs	Fibre	kJ/Cal
Breakfast 1 2 3 4 5 ○ ○ ○ ○ ○ HUNGER SCALE								
Mid-morning ○ ○ ○ ○ ○								
Lunch 1 2 3 4 5 ○ ○ ○ ○ ○ HUNGER SCALE								
Mid-afternoon ○ ○ ○ ○ ○								
Dinner 1 2 3 4 5 ○ ○ ○ ○ ○ HUNGER SCALE								
Evening ○ ○ ○ ○ ○								

Coffees/teas   Fluid intake ▽▽▽▽▽▽▽▽▽▽   Daily totals

THURSDAY

	Time		Quantity	Fat	Protein	Carbs	Fibre	kJ/Cal
Breakfast 1 2 3 4 5 ○ ○ ○ ○ ○ HUNGER SCALE								
Mid-morning ○ ○ ○ ○ ○								
Lunch 1 2 3 4 5 ○ ○ ○ ○ ○ HUNGER SCALE								
Mid-afternoon ○ ○ ○ ○ ○								
Dinner 1 2 3 4 5 ○ ○ ○ ○ ○ HUNGER SCALE								
Evening ○ ○ ○ ○ ○								

Coffees/teas   Fluid intake ▽▽▽▽▽▽▽▽▽▽   Daily totals

FRIDAY

	Time		Quantity	Fat	Protein	Carbs	Fibre	kJ/Cal
Breakfast 1 2 3 4 5 ○ ○ ○ ○ ○ HUNGER SCALE								
Mid-morning ○ ○ ○ ○ ○								
Lunch 1 2 3 4 5 ○ ○ ○ ○ ○ HUNGER SCALE								
Mid-afternoon ○ ○ ○ ○ ○								
Dinner 1 2 3 4 5 ○ ○ ○ ○ ○ HUNGER SCALE								
Evening ○ ○ ○ ○ ○								

Coffees/teas   Fluid intake ▽▽▽▽▽▽▽▽▽▽   Daily totals

SATURDAY

	Time					Quantity	Fat	Protein	Carbs	Fibre	kJ/Cal
Breakfast 1 2 3 4 5 ○○○○○ HUNGER SCALE											
Mid-morning ○○○○○											
Lunch 1 2 3 4 5 ○○○○○ HUNGER SCALE											
Mid-afternoon ○○○○○											
Dinner 1 2 3 4 5 ○○○○○ HUNGER SCALE											
Evening ○○○○○											

Coffees/teas [ ]　Fluid intake ⊔⊔⊔⊔⊔⊔⊔⊔⊔⊔　Daily totals

SUNDAY

						Quantity	Fat	Protein	Carbs	Fibre	kJ/Cal
Breakfast 1 2 3 4 5 ○○○○○ HUNGER SCALE											
Mid-morning ○○○○○											
Lunch 1 2 3 4 5 ○○○○○ HUNGER SCALE											
Mid-afternoon ○○○○○											
Dinner 1 2 3 4 5 ○○○○○ HUNGER SCALE											
Evening ○○○○○											

Coffees/teas [ ]　Fluid intake ⊔⊔⊔⊔⊔⊔⊔⊔⊔⊔　Daily totals

Units of alcohol this week [ ]　**Total alcohol kJ/Cal** [ ]

Vitamins and supplements

	Fat	Protein	Carbs	Fibre	kJ/Cal
WEEKLY TOTALS					

WEEKLY PERSONAL SUMMARY

Mood 1 2 3 4 5 ○○○○○　**Appetite** 1 2 3 4 5 ○○○○○

Energy level 1 2 3 4 5 ○○○○○　**Stress level** 1 2 3 4 5 ○○○○○

Hours of sleep [ ]　**Sleep quality** 1 2 3 4 5 ○○○○○

Injuries or illnesses [ ]

kJ/Cal intake

Planned kJ/Cal	
Actual kJ/Cal	
Difference [+/-]	

Weight at end of week [ ]

BMI at end of week [ ]

EXERCISE DIARY

STRENGTH TRAINING		SET 1		SET 2		SET 3		SET4			
Exercise	Focus area	Reps	Weight	Reps	Weight	Reps	Weight	Reps	Weight	Equipment	Ease

CARDIO TRAINING

Exercise	Time	Distance	Intensity	Heart rate	Ease	kJ/Cal burnt

Total kJ/Cal burnt

INCIDENTAL EXERCISE

Day	Activity	Day	Activity

WEEK BEGINNING   /   /

Weight at start of week

BMI at start of week

Planned kJ/Cal this week

Possible diet-busting occasions this week

Planned exercise sessions this week

	Exercise	Completed [Y/N]
Monday		
Tuesday		
Wednesday		
Thursday		
Friday		
Saturday		
Sunday		

FOOD DIARY

MONDAY

	Time		Quantity	Fat	Protein	Carbs	Fibre	kJ/Cal
Breakfast 1 2 3 4 5 ○○○○○ HUNGER SCALE								
Mid-morning ○○○○○								
Lunch 1 2 3 4 5 ○○○○○ HUNGER SCALE								
Mid-afternoon ○○○○○								
Dinner 1 2 3 4 5 ○○○○○ HUNGER SCALE								
Evening ○○○○○								

Coffees/teas   Fluid intake ⎕⎕⎕⎕⎕⎕⎕⎕⎕⎕   Daily totals

TUESDAY

	Time		Quantity	Fat	Protein	Carbs	Fibre	kJ/Cal
Breakfast 1 2 3 4 5 ○○○○○ HUNGER SCALE								
Mid-morning ○○○○○								
Lunch 1 2 3 4 5 ○○○○○ HUNGER SCALE								
Mid-afternoon ○○○○○								
Dinner 1 2 3 4 5 ○○○○○ HUNGER SCALE								
Evening ○○○○○								

Coffees/teas   Fluid intake ⎕⎕⎕⎕⎕⎕⎕⎕⎕⎕   Daily totals

WEDNESDAY	Time		Quantity	Fat	Protein	Carbs	Fibre	kJ/Cal
Breakfast 1 2 3 4 5 ○ ○ ○ ○ ○ HUNGER SCALE								
Mid-morning ○ ○ ○ ○ ○								
Lunch 1 2 3 4 5 ○ ○ ○ ○ ○ HUNGER SCALE								
Mid-afternoon ○ ○ ○ ○ ○								
Dinner 1 2 3 4 5 ○ ○ ○ ○ ○ HUNGER SCALE								
Evening ○ ○ ○ ○ ○								
Coffees/teas		Fluid intake ⎕⎕⎕⎕⎕⎕⎕⎕⎕⎕	Daily totals					

THURSDAY								
Breakfast 1 2 3 4 5 ○ ○ ○ ○ ○ HUNGER SCALE								
Mid-morning ○ ○ ○ ○ ○								
Lunch 1 2 3 4 5 ○ ○ ○ ○ ○ HUNGER SCALE								
Mid-afternoon ○ ○ ○ ○ ○								
Dinner 1 2 3 4 5 ○ ○ ○ ○ ○ HUNGER SCALE								
Evening ○ ○ ○ ○ ○								
Coffees/teas		Fluid intake ⎕⎕⎕⎕⎕⎕⎕⎕⎕⎕	Daily totals					

FRIDAY								
Breakfast 1 2 3 4 5 ○ ○ ○ ○ ○ HUNGER SCALE								
Mid-morning ○ ○ ○ ○ ○								
Lunch 1 2 3 4 5 ○ ○ ○ ○ ○ HUNGER SCALE								
Mid-afternoon ○ ○ ○ ○ ○								
Dinner 1 2 3 4 5 ○ ○ ○ ○ ○ HUNGER SCALE								
Evening ○ ○ ○ ○ ○								
Coffees/teas		Fluid intake ⎕⎕⎕⎕⎕⎕⎕⎕⎕⎕	Daily totals					

SATURDAY

	Time							Quantity	Fat	Protein	Carbs	Fibre	kJ/Cal
Breakfast 1 2 3 4 5 ○○○○○ HUNGER SCALE													
Mid-morning ○○○○○													
Lunch 1 2 3 4 5 ○○○○○ HUNGER SCALE													
Mid-afternoon ○○○○○													
Dinner 1 2 3 4 5 ○○○○○ HUNGER SCALE													
Evening ○○○○○													

Coffees/teas ☐   Fluid intake ▽▽▽▽▽▽▽▽▽▽   Daily totals

SUNDAY

	Time							Quantity	Fat	Protein	Carbs	Fibre	kJ/Cal
Breakfast 1 2 3 4 5 ○○○○○ HUNGER SCALE													
Mid-morning ○○○○○													
Lunch 1 2 3 4 5 ○○○○○ HUNGER SCALE													
Mid-afternoon ○○○○○													
Dinner 1 2 3 4 5 ○○○○○ HUNGER SCALE													
Evening ○○○○○													

Coffees/teas ☐   Fluid intake ▽▽▽▽▽▽▽▽▽▽   Daily totals

Units of alcohol this week ☐   Total alcohol kJ/Cal ☐

Vitamins and supplements

	Fat	Protein	Carbs	Fibre	kJ/Cal
WEEKLY TOTALS					

WEEKLY PERSONAL SUMMARY

Mood 1 2 3 4 5 ○○○○○   **Appetite** 1 2 3 4 5 ○○○○○

Energy level 1 2 3 4 5 ○○○○○   **Stress level** 1 2 3 4 5 ○○○○○

Hours of sleep ☐   **Sleep quality** 1 2 3 4 5 ○○○○○

kJ/Cal intake	
Planned kJ/Cal	
Actual kJ/Cal	
Difference [+/-]	

Weight at end of week

BMI at end of week

Injuries or illnesses

EXERCISE DIARY

STRENGTH TRAINING		SET 1		SET 2		SET 3		SET4			
Exercise	Focus area	Reps	Weight	Reps	Weight	Reps	Weight	Reps	Weight	Equipment	Ease

CARDIO TRAINING

Exercise	Time	Distance	Intensity	Heart rate	Ease	kJ/Cal burnt

Total kJ/Cal burnt

INCIDENTAL EXERCISE

Day	Activity	Day	Activity

WEEK BEGINNING   /   /

Weight at start of week

BMI at start of week

Planned kJ/Cal this week

Possible diet-busting occasions this week

Planned exercise sessions this week

	Exercise	Completed [Y/N]
Monday		
Tuesday		
Wednesday		
Thursday		
Friday		
Saturday		
Sunday		

FOOD DIARY

MONDAY

	Time		Quantity	Fat	Protein	Carbs	Fibre	kJ/Cal
Breakfast 1 2 3 4 5 ○ ○ ○ ○ ○ HUNGER SCALE								
Mid-morning ○ ○ ○ ○ ○								
Lunch 1 2 3 4 5 ○ ○ ○ ○ ○ HUNGER SCALE								
Mid-afternoon ○ ○ ○ ○ ○								
Dinner 1 2 3 4 5 ○ ○ ○ ○ ○ HUNGER SCALE								
Evening ○ ○ ○ ○ ○								

Coffees/teas   Fluid intake ▽▽▽▽▽▽▽▽▽▽   Daily totals

TUESDAY

Breakfast 1 2 3 4 5 ○ ○ ○ ○ ○ HUNGER SCALE								
Mid-morning ○ ○ ○ ○ ○								
Lunch 1 2 3 4 5 ○ ○ ○ ○ ○ HUNGER SCALE								
Mid-afternoon ○ ○ ○ ○ ○								
Dinner 1 2 3 4 5 ○ ○ ○ ○ ○ HUNGER SCALE								
Evening ○ ○ ○ ○ ○								

Coffees/teas   Fluid intake ▽▽▽▽▽▽▽▽▽▽   Daily totals

WEDNESDAY

	Time		Quantity	Fat	Protein	Carbs	Fibre	kJ/Cal
Breakfast 1 2 3 4 5 ○○○○○ HUNGER SCALE								
Mid-morning ○○○○○								
Lunch 1 2 3 4 5 ○○○○○ HUNGER SCALE								
Mid-afternoon ○○○○○								
Dinner 1 2 3 4 5 ○○○○○ HUNGER SCALE								
Evening ○○○○○								

Coffees/teas ☐   Fluid intake 🥛🥛🥛🥛🥛🥛🥛🥛🥛🥛   Daily totals

THURSDAY

	Time		Quantity	Fat	Protein	Carbs	Fibre	kJ/Cal
Breakfast 1 2 3 4 5 ○○○○○ HUNGER SCALE								
Mid-morning ○○○○○								
Lunch 1 2 3 4 5 ○○○○○ HUNGER SCALE								
Mid-afternoon ○○○○○								
Dinner 1 2 3 4 5 ○○○○○ HUNGER SCALE								
Evening ○○○○○								

Coffees/teas ☐   Fluid intake 🥛🥛🥛🥛🥛🥛🥛🥛🥛🥛   Daily totals

FRIDAY

	Time		Quantity	Fat	Protein	Carbs	Fibre	kJ/Cal
Breakfast 1 2 3 4 5 ○○○○○ HUNGER SCALE								
Mid-morning ○○○○○								
Lunch 1 2 3 4 5 ○○○○○ HUNGER SCALE								
Mid-afternoon ○○○○○								
Dinner 1 2 3 4 5 ○○○○○ HUNGER SCALE								
Evening ○○○○○								

Coffees/teas ☐   Fluid intake 🥛🥛🥛🥛🥛🥛🥛🥛🥛🥛   Daily totals

SATURDAY

	Time			Quantity	Fat	Protein	Carbs	Fibre	kJ/Cal
Breakfast 1 2 3 4 5 ○○○○○ HUNGER SCALE									
Mid-morning ○○○○○									
Lunch 1 2 3 4 5 ○○○○○ HUNGER SCALE									
Mid-afternoon ○○○○○									
Dinner 1 2 3 4 5 ○○○○○ HUNGER SCALE									
Evening ○○○○○									

Coffees/teas ☐   Fluid intake ▽▽▽▽▽▽▽▽▽▽   Daily totals

SUNDAY

					Fat	Protein	Carbs	Fibre	kJ/Cal
Breakfast 1 2 3 4 5 ○○○○○ HUNGER SCALE									
Mid-morning ○○○○○									
Lunch 1 2 3 4 5 ○○○○○ HUNGER SCALE									
Mid-afternoon ○○○○○									
Dinner 1 2 3 4 5 ○○○○○ HUNGER SCALE									
Evening ○○○○○									

Coffees/teas ☐   Fluid intake ▽▽▽▽▽▽▽▽▽▽   Daily totals

Units of alcohol this week ☐   Total alcohol kJ/Cal

Vitamins and supplements

WEEKLY TOTALS	Fat	Protein	Carbs	Fibre	kJ/Cal

WEEKLY PERSONAL SUMMARY

Mood 1 2 3 4 5 ○○○○○   **Appetite** 1 2 3 4 5 ○○○○○

Energy level 1 2 3 4 5 ○○○○○   **Stress level** 1 2 3 4 5 ○○○○○

Hours of sleep ☐   **Sleep quality** 1 2 3 4 5 ○○○○○

Injuries or illnesses

kJ/Cal intake	
Planned kJ/Cal	
Actual kJ/Cal	
Difference [+/-]	

Weight at end of week ☐

BMI at end of week ☐

EXERCISE DIARY

STRENGTH TRAINING		SET 1		SET 2		SET 3		SET4			
Exercise	Focus area	Reps	Weight	Reps	Weight	Reps	Weight	Reps	Weight	Equipment	Ease

CARDIO TRAINING

Exercise	Time	Distance	Intensity	Heart rate	Ease	kJ/Cal burnt

Total kJ/Cal burnt

INCIDENTAL EXERCISE

Day	Activity	Day	Activity

WEEK BEGINNING   /   /

Weight at start of week

BMI at start of week

Planned kJ/Cal this week

Possible diet-busting occasions this week

Planned exercise sessions this week

	Exercise	Completed [Y/N]
Monday		
Tuesday		
Wednesday		
Thursday		
Friday		
Saturday		
Sunday		

FOOD DIARY

MONDAY

	Time		Quantity	Fat	Protein	Carbs	Fibre	kJ/Cal
Breakfast 1 2 3 4 5 ○○○○○ HUNGER SCALE								
Mid-morning ○○○○○								
Lunch 1 2 3 4 5 ○○○○○ HUNGER SCALE								
Mid-afternoon ○○○○○								
Dinner 1 2 3 4 5 ○○○○○ HUNGER SCALE								
Evening ○○○○○								

Coffees/teas   Fluid intake ▽▽▽▽▽▽▽▽▽▽   Daily totals

TUESDAY

	Time		Quantity	Fat	Protein	Carbs	Fibre	kJ/Cal
Breakfast 1 2 3 4 5 ○○○○○ HUNGER SCALE								
Mid-morning ○○○○○								
Lunch 1 2 3 4 5 ○○○○○ HUNGER SCALE								
Mid-afternoon ○○○○○								
Dinner 1 2 3 4 5 ○○○○○ HUNGER SCALE								
Evening ○○○○○								

Coffees/teas   Fluid intake ▽▽▽▽▽▽▽▽▽▽   Daily totals

WEDNESDAY

	Time		Quantity	Fat	Protein	Carbs	Fibre	kJ/Cal
Breakfast 1 2 3 4 5 ○○○○ HUNGER SCALE								
Mid-morning ○○○○○								
Lunch 1 2 3 4 5 ○○○○○ HUNGER SCALE								
Mid-afternoon ○○○○○								
Dinner 1 2 3 4 5 ○○○○○ HUNGER SCALE								
Evening ○○○○○								

Coffees/teas　　　Fluid intake ▽▽▽▽▽▽▽▽▽▽　　Daily totals

THURSDAY

	Time		Quantity	Fat	Protein	Carbs	Fibre	kJ/Cal
Breakfast 1 2 3 4 5 ○○○○○ HUNGER SCALE								
Mid-morning ○○○○○								
Lunch 1 2 3 4 5 ○○○○○ HUNGER SCALE								
Mid-afternoon ○○○○○								
Dinner 1 2 3 4 5 ○○○○○ HUNGER SCALE								
Evening ○○○○○								

Coffees/teas　　　Fluid intake ▽▽▽▽▽▽▽▽▽▽　　Daily totals

FRIDAY

	Time		Quantity	Fat	Protein	Carbs	Fibre	kJ/Cal
Breakfast 1 2 3 4 5 ○○○○○ HUNGER SCALE								
Mid-morning ○○○○○								
Lunch 1 2 3 4 5 ○○○○○ HUNGER SCALE								
Mid-afternoon ○○○○○								
Dinner 1 2 3 4 5 ○○○○○ HUNGER SCALE								
Evening ○○○○○								

Coffees/teas　　　Fluid intake ▽▽▽▽▽▽▽▽▽▽　　Daily totals

SATURDAY

	Time							Quantity	Fat	Protein	Carbs	Fibre	kJ/Cal
Breakfast 1 2 3 4 5 ○ ○ ○ ○ ○ HUNGER SCALE													
Mid-morning ○ ○ ○ ○ ○													
Lunch 1 2 3 4 5 ○ ○ ○ ○ ○ HUNGER SCALE													
Mid-afternoon ○ ○ ○ ○ ○													
Dinner 1 2 3 4 5 ○ ○ ○ ○ ○ HUNGER SCALE													
Evening ○ ○ ○ ○ ○													

Coffees/teas ▢ Fluid intake ▯▯▯▯▯▯▯▯▯▯ Daily totals

SUNDAY

	Time							Quantity	Fat	Protein	Carbs	Fibre	kJ/Cal
Breakfast 1 2 3 4 5 ○ ○ ○ ○ ○ HUNGER SCALE													
Mid-morning ○ ○ ○ ○ ○													
Lunch 1 2 3 4 5 ○ ○ ○ ○ ○ HUNGER SCALE													
Mid-afternoon ○ ○ ○ ○ ○													
Dinner 1 2 3 4 5 ○ ○ ○ ○ ○ HUNGER SCALE													
Evening ○ ○ ○ ○ ○													

Coffees/teas ▢ Fluid intake ▯▯▯▯▯▯▯▯▯▯ Daily totals

Units of alcohol this week ▢ **Total alcohol kJ/Cal** ▢

Vitamins and supplements

WEEKLY TOTALS	Fat	Protein	Carbs	Fibre	kJ/Cal

WEEKLY PERSONAL SUMMARY

Mood 1 2 3 4 5 ○ ○ ○ ○ ○   **Appetite** 1 2 3 4 5 ○ ○ ○ ○ ○

Energy level 1 2 3 4 5 ○ ○ ○ ○ ○   **Stress level** 1 2 3 4 5 ○ ○ ○ ○ ○

Hours of sleep ▢   **Sleep quality** 1 2 3 4 5 ○ ○ ○ ○ ○

Injuries or illnesses

kJ/Cal intake

Planned kJ/Cal	
Actual kJ/Cal	

Difference [+/-]

Weight at end of week

BMI at end of week

EXERCISE DIARY

STRENGTH TRAINING		SET 1		SET 2		SET 3		SET4			
Exercise	Focus area	Reps	Weight	Reps	Weight	Reps	Weight	Reps	Weight	Equipment	Ease

CARDIO TRAINING

Exercise	Time	Distance	Intensity	Heart rate	Ease	kJ/Cal burnt

Total kJ/Cal burnt

INCIDENTAL EXERCISE

Day	Activity	Day	Activity

WEEK BEGINNING   /   /

Weight at start of week

BMI at start of week

Planned kJ/Cal this week

Possible diet-busting occasions this week

Planned exercise sessions this week

	Exercise	Completed [Y/N]
Monday		
Tuesday		
Wednesday		
Thursday		
Friday		
Saturday		
Sunday		

FOOD DIARY

MONDAY

	Time		Quantity	Fat	Protein	Carbs	Fibre	kJ/Cal
Breakfast 1 2 3 4 5 ○ ○ ○ ○ ○ HUNGER SCALE								
Mid-morning ○ ○ ○ ○ ○								
Lunch 1 2 3 4 5 ○ ○ ○ ○ ○ HUNGER SCALE								
Mid-afternoon ○ ○ ○ ○ ○								
Dinner 1 2 3 4 5 ○ ○ ○ ○ ○ HUNGER SCALE								
Evening ○ ○ ○ ○								

Coffees/teas   Fluid intake ▽▽▽▽▽▽▽▽▽▽   Daily totals

TUESDAY

	Time		Quantity	Fat	Protein	Carbs	Fibre	kJ/Cal
Breakfast 1 2 3 4 5 ○ ○ ○ ○ ○ HUNGER SCALE								
Mid-morning ○ ○ ○ ○ ○								
Lunch 1 2 3 4 5 ○ ○ ○ ○ ○ HUNGER SCALE								
Mid-afternoon ○ ○ ○ ○ ○								
Dinner 1 2 3 4 5 ○ ○ ○ ○ ○ HUNGER SCALE								
Evening ○ ○ ○ ○								

Coffees/teas   Fluid intake ▽▽▽▽▽▽▽▽▽▽   Daily totals

WEDNESDAY

	Time			Quantity	Fat	Protein	Carbs	Fibre	kJ/Cal
Breakfast 1 2 3 4 5 ○ ○ ○ ○ ○ HUNGER SCALE									
Mid-morning ○ ○ ○ ○ ○									
Lunch 1 2 3 4 5 ○ ○ ○ ○ ○ HUNGER SCALE									
Mid-afternoon ○ ○ ○ ○ ○									
Dinner 1 2 3 4 5 ○ ○ ○ ○ ○ HUNGER SCALE									
Evening ○ ○ ○ ○ ○									

Coffees/teas ▢ Fluid intake ⬭⬭⬭⬭⬭⬭⬭⬭⬭⬭ Daily totals

THURSDAY

	Time			Quantity	Fat	Protein	Carbs	Fibre	kJ/Cal
Breakfast 1 2 3 4 5 ○ ○ ○ ○ ○ HUNGER SCALE									
Mid-morning ○ ○ ○ ○ ○									
Lunch 1 2 3 4 5 ○ ○ ○ ○ ○ HUNGER SCALE									
Mid-afternoon ○ ○ ○ ○ ○									
Dinner 1 2 3 4 5 ○ ○ ○ ○ ○ HUNGER SCALE									
Evening ○ ○ ○ ○ ○									

Coffees/teas ▢ Fluid intake ⬭⬭⬭⬭⬭⬭⬭⬭⬭⬭ Daily totals

FRIDAY

	Time			Quantity	Fat	Protein	Carbs	Fibre	kJ/Cal
Breakfast 1 2 3 4 5 ○ ○ ○ ○ ○ HUNGER SCALE									
Mid-morning ○ ○ ○ ○ ○									
Lunch 1 2 3 4 5 ○ ○ ○ ○ ○ HUNGER SCALE									
Mid-afternoon ○ ○ ○ ○ ○									
Dinner 1 2 3 4 5 ○ ○ ○ ○ ○ HUNGER SCALE									
Evening ○ ○ ○ ○ ○									

Coffees/teas ▢ Fluid intake ⬭⬭⬭⬭⬭⬭⬭⬭⬭⬭ Daily totals

SATURDAY

	Time		Quantity	Fat	Protein	Carbs	Fibre	kJ/Cal
Breakfast 1 2 3 4 5 ○○○○○ HUNGER SCALE								
Mid-morning ○○○○○								
Lunch 1 2 3 4 5 ○○○○○ HUNGER SCALE								
Mid-afternoon ○○○○○								
Dinner 1 2 3 4 5 ○○○○○ HUNGER SCALE								
Evening ○○○○○								

Coffees/teas [   ]   Fluid intake ▭▭▭▭▭▭▭▭▭▭   Daily totals

SUNDAY

	Time		Quantity	Fat	Protein	Carbs	Fibre	kJ/Cal
Breakfast 1 2 3 4 5 ○○○○○ HUNGER SCALE								
Mid-morning ○○○○○								
Lunch 1 2 3 4 5 ○○○○○ HUNGER SCALE								
Mid-afternoon ○○○○○								
Dinner 1 2 3 4 5 ○○○○○ HUNGER SCALE								
Evening ○○○○○								

Coffees/teas [   ]   Fluid intake ▭▭▭▭▭▭▭▭▭▭   Daily totals

Units of alcohol this week [   ]   Total alcohol kJ/Cal [   ]

Vitamins and supplements

	Fat	Protein	Carbs	Fibre	kJ/Cal
WEEKLY TOTALS					

WEEKLY PERSONAL SUMMARY

Mood 1 2 3 4 5 ○○○○○   **Appetite** 1 2 3 4 5 ○○○○○

Energy level 1 2 3 4 5 ○○○○○   **Stress level** 1 2 3 4 5 ○○○○○

Hours of sleep [   ]   **Sleep quality** 1 2 3 4 5 ○○○○○

kJ/Cal intake

Planned kJ/Cal	
Actual kJ/Cal	
Difference [+/-]	

Weight at end of week [   ]

BMI at end of week

Injuries or illnesses

EXERCISE DIARY

STRENGTH TRAINING		SET 1		SET 2		SET 3		SET4			
Exercise	Focus area	Reps	Weight	Reps	Weight	Reps	Weight	Reps	Weight	Equipment	Ease

CARDIO TRAINING

Exercise	Time	Distance	Intensity	Heart rate	Ease	kJ/Cal burnt

Total kJ/Cal burnt

INCIDENTAL EXERCISE

Day	Activity	Day	Activity

WEEK BEGINNING   /   /

Weight at start of week

BMI at start of week

Planned kJ/Cal this week

Possible diet-busting occasions this week

Planned exercise sessions this week

	Exercise	Completed [Y/N]
Monday		
Tuesday		
Wednesday		
Thursday		
Friday		
Saturday		
Sunday		

FOOD DIARY

MONDAY

	Time		Quantity	Fat	Protein	Carbs	Fibre	kJ/Cal
Breakfast 1 2 3 4 5 ○ ○ ○ ○ ○ HUNGER SCALE								
Mid-morning ○ ○ ○ ○ ○								
Lunch 1 2 3 4 5 ○ ○ ○ ○ ○ HUNGER SCALE								
Mid-afternoon ○ ○ ○ ○ ○								
Dinner 1 2 3 4 5 ○ ○ ○ ○ ○ HUNGER SCALE								
Evening ○ ○ ○ ○ ○								

Coffees/teas   Fluid intake ☐ ☐ ☐ ☐ ☐ ☐ ☐ ☐ ☐ ☐   Daily totals

TUESDAY

			Quantity	Fat	Protein	Carbs	Fibre	kJ/Cal
Breakfast 1 2 3 4 5 ○ ○ ○ ○ ○ HUNGER SCALE								
Mid-morning ○ ○ ○ ○ ○								
Lunch 1 2 3 4 5 ○ ○ ○ ○ ○ HUNGER SCALE								
Mid-afternoon ○ ○ ○ ○ ○								
Dinner 1 2 3 4 5 ○ ○ ○ ○ ○ HUNGER SCALE								
Evening ○ ○ ○ ○ ○								

Coffees/teas   Fluid intake ☐ ☐ ☐ ☐ ☐ ☐ ☐ ☐ ☐ ☐   Daily totals

WEDNESDAY

	Time		Quantity	Fat	Protein	Carbs	Fibre	kJ/Cal
Breakfast 1 2 3 4 5 ○○○○○ HUNGER SCALE								
Mid-morning ○○○○○								
Lunch 1 2 3 4 5 ○○○○○ HUNGER SCALE								
Mid-afternoon ○○○○○								
Dinner 1 2 3 4 5 ○○○○○ HUNGER SCALE								
Evening ○○○○○								

Coffees/teas   Fluid intake ⛾⛾⛾⛾⛾⛾⛾⛾⛾⛾   Daily totals

THURSDAY

	Time		Quantity	Fat	Protein	Carbs	Fibre	kJ/Cal
Breakfast 1 2 3 4 5 ○○○○○ HUNGER SCALE								
Mid-morning ○○○○○								
Lunch 1 2 3 4 5 ○○○○○ HUNGER SCALE								
Mid-afternoon ○○○○○								
Dinner 1 2 3 4 5 ○○○○○ HUNGER SCALE								
Evening ○○○○○								

Coffees/teas   Fluid intake ⛾⛾⛾⛾⛾⛾⛾⛾⛾⛾   Daily totals

FRIDAY

	Time		Quantity	Fat	Protein	Carbs	Fibre	kJ/Cal
Breakfast 1 2 3 4 5 ○○○○○ HUNGER SCALE								
Mid-morning ○○○○○								
Lunch 1 2 3 4 5 ○○○○○ HUNGER SCALE								
Mid-afternoon ○○○○○								
Dinner 1 2 3 4 5 ○○○○○ HUNGER SCALE								
Evening ○○○○○								

Coffees/teas   Fluid intake ⛾⛾⛾⛾⛾⛾⛾⛾⛾⛾   Daily totals

SATURDAY

	Time		Quantity	Fat	Protein	Carbs	Fibre	kJ/Cal
Breakfast 1 2 3 4 5 ○○○○○ HUNGER SCALE								
Mid-morning ○○○○○								
Lunch 1 2 3 4 5 ○○○○○ HUNGER SCALE								
Mid-afternoon ○○○○○								
Dinner 1 2 3 4 5 ○○○○○ HUNGER SCALE								
Evening ○○○○○								

Coffees/teas ▢   Fluid intake ▢▢▢▢▢▢▢▢▢▢   Daily totals

SUNDAY

	Time		Quantity	Fat	Protein	Carbs	Fibre	kJ/Cal
Breakfast 1 2 3 4 5 ○○○○○ HUNGER SCALE								
Mid-morning ○○○○○								
Lunch 1 2 3 4 5 ○○○○○ HUNGER SCALE								
Mid-afternoon ○○○○○								
Dinner 1 2 3 4 5 ○○○○○ HUNGER SCALE								
Evening ○○○○○								

Coffees/teas ▢   Fluid intake ▢▢▢▢▢▢▢▢▢▢   Daily totals

Units of alcohol this week   **Total alcohol kJ/Cal**

Vitamins and supplements

WEEKLY TOTALS	Fat	Protein	Carbs	Fibre	kJ/Cal

WEEKLY PERSONAL SUMMARY

Mood 1 2 3 4 5 ○○○○○   **Appetite** 1 2 3 4 5 ○○○○○

Energy level 1 2 3 4 5 ○○○○○   **Stress level** 1 2 3 4 5 ○○○○○

Hours of sleep   **Sleep quality** 1 2 3 4 5 ○○○○○

kJ/Cal intake

Planned kJ/Cal	
Actual kJ/Cal	
Difference [+/-]	

Weight at end of week

BMI at end of week

Injuries or illnesses

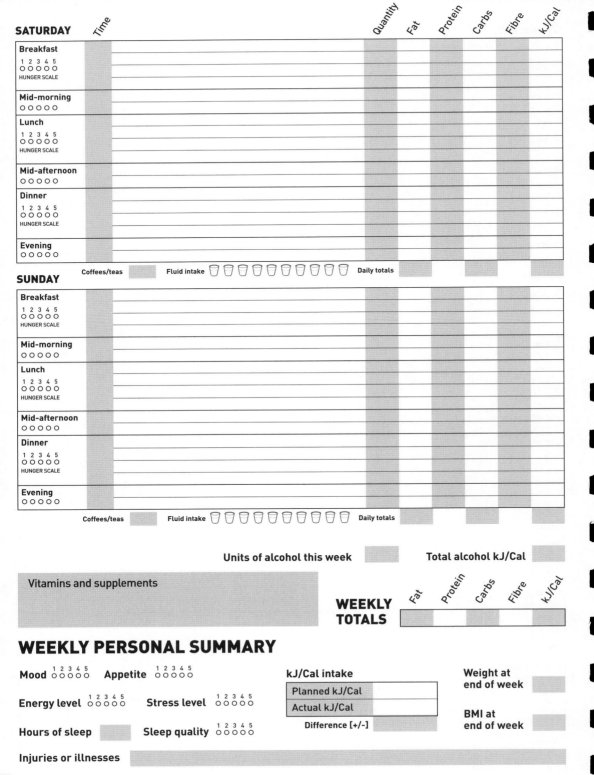

EXERCISE DIARY

STRENGTH TRAINING		SET 1		SET 2		SET 3		SET 4			
Exercise	Focus area	Reps	Weight	Reps	Weight	Reps	Weight	Reps	Weight	Equipment	Ease

CARDIO TRAINING

Exercise	Time	Distance	Intensity	Heart rate	Ease	kJ/Cal burnt

Total kJ/Cal burnt

INCIDENTAL EXERCISE

Day	Activity	Day	Activity

WEEK BEGINNING / /

Weight at start of week

BMI at start of week

Planned kJ/Cal this week

Possible diet-busting occasions this week

Planned exercise sessions this week

	Exercise	Completed [Y/N]
Monday		
Tuesday		
Wednesday		
Thursday		
Friday		
Saturday		
Sunday		

FOOD DIARY

MONDAY

	Time		Quantity	Fat	Protein	Carbs	Fibre	kJ/Cal
Breakfast 1 2 3 4 5 ○ ○ ○ ○ ○ HUNGER SCALE								
Mid-morning ○ ○ ○ ○ ○								
Lunch 1 2 3 4 5 ○ ○ ○ ○ ○ HUNGER SCALE								
Mid-afternoon ○ ○ ○ ○ ○								
Dinner 1 2 3 4 5 ○ ○ ○ ○ ○ HUNGER SCALE								
Evening ○ ○ ○ ○ ○								

Coffees/teas   Fluid intake ▽▽▽▽▽▽▽▽▽▽   Daily totals

TUESDAY

	Time		Quantity	Fat	Protein	Carbs	Fibre	kJ/Cal
Breakfast 1 2 3 4 5 ○ ○ ○ ○ ○ HUNGER SCALE								
Mid-morning ○ ○ ○ ○ ○								
Lunch 1 2 3 4 5 ○ ○ ○ ○ ○ HUNGER SCALE								
Mid-afternoon ○ ○ ○ ○ ○								
Dinner 1 2 3 4 5 ○ ○ ○ ○ ○ HUNGER SCALE								
Evening ○ ○ ○ ○ ○								

Coffees/teas   Fluid intake ▽▽▽▽▽▽▽▽▽▽   Daily totals

WEDNESDAY

	Time		Quantity	Fat	Protein	Carbs	Fibre	kJ/Cal
Breakfast 1 2 3 4 5 ○○○○○ HUNGER SCALE								
Mid-morning ○○○○○								
Lunch 1 2 3 4 5 ○○○○○ HUNGER SCALE								
Mid-afternoon ○○○○○								
Dinner 1 2 3 4 5 ○○○○○ HUNGER SCALE								
Evening ○○○○○								

Coffees/teas ▭ Fluid intake ▭▭▭▭▭▭▭▭▭▭ Daily totals

THURSDAY

Breakfast 1 2 3 4 5 ○○○○○ HUNGER SCALE								
Mid-morning ○○○○○								
Lunch 1 2 3 4 5 ○○○○○ HUNGER SCALE								
Mid-afternoon ○○○○○								
Dinner 1 2 3 4 5 ○○○○○ HUNGER SCALE								
Evening ○○○○○								

Coffees/teas ▭ Fluid intake ▭▭▭▭▭▭▭▭▭▭ Daily totals

FRIDAY

Breakfast 1 2 3 4 5 ○○○○○ HUNGER SCALE								
Mid-morning ○○○○○								
Lunch 1 2 3 4 5 ○○○○○ HUNGER SCALE								
Mid-afternoon ○○○○○								
Dinner 1 2 3 4 5 ○○○○○ HUNGER SCALE								
Evening ○○○○○								

Coffees/teas ▭ Fluid intake ▭▭▭▭▭▭▭▭▭▭ Daily totals

SATURDAY

	Time							Quantity	Fat	Protein	Carbs	Fibre	kJ/Cal
Breakfast 1 2 3 4 5 ○ ○ ○ ○ ○ HUNGER SCALE													
Mid-morning ○ ○ ○ ○ ○													
Lunch 1 2 3 4 5 ○ ○ ○ ○ ○ HUNGER SCALE													
Mid-afternoon ○ ○ ○ ○ ○													
Dinner 1 2 3 4 5 ○ ○ ○ ○ ○ HUNGER SCALE													
Evening ○ ○ ○ ○ ○													

Coffees/teas   Fluid intake ▽▽▽▽▽▽▽▽▽▽   Daily totals

SUNDAY

	Time							Quantity	Fat	Protein	Carbs	Fibre	kJ/Cal
Breakfast 1 2 3 4 5 ○ ○ ○ ○ ○ HUNGER SCALE													
Mid-morning ○ ○ ○ ○ ○													
Lunch 1 2 3 4 5 ○ ○ ○ ○ ○ HUNGER SCALE													
Mid-afternoon ○ ○ ○ ○ ○													
Dinner 1 2 3 4 5 ○ ○ ○ ○ ○ HUNGER SCALE													
Evening ○ ○ ○ ○ ○													

Coffees/teas   Fluid intake ▽▽▽▽▽▽▽▽▽▽   Daily totals

Units of alcohol this week   **Total alcohol kJ/Cal**

Vitamins and supplements

	Fat	Protein	Carbs	Fibre	kJ/Cal
WEEKLY TOTALS					

WEEKLY PERSONAL SUMMARY

Mood 1 2 3 4 5 ○ ○ ○ ○ ○   **Appetite** 1 2 3 4 5 ○ ○ ○ ○ ○

Energy level 1 2 3 4 5 ○ ○ ○ ○ ○   **Stress level** 1 2 3 4 5 ○ ○ ○ ○ ○

Hours of sleep   **Sleep quality** 1 2 3 4 5 ○ ○ ○ ○ ○

Injuries or illnesses

kJ/Cal intake

Planned kJ/Cal	
Actual kJ/Cal	
Difference [+/-]	

Weight at end of week

BMI at end of week

EXERCISE DIARY

STRENGTH TRAINING		SET 1		SET 2		SET 3		SET4			
Exercise	Focus area	Reps	Weight	Reps	Weight	Reps	Weight	Reps	Weight	Equipment	Ease

CARDIO TRAINING

Exercise	Time	Distance	Intensity	Heart rate	Ease	kJ/Cal burnt

Total kJ/Cal burnt

INCIDENTAL EXERCISE

Day	Activity	Day	Activity

WEEK BEGINNING / /

Weight at start of week

BMI at start of week

Planned kJ/Cal this week

Possible diet-busting occasions this week

Planned exercise sessions this week

	Exercise	Completed [Y/N]
Monday		
Tuesday		
Wednesday		
Thursday		
Friday		
Saturday		
Sunday		

FOOD DIARY

MONDAY

	Time		Quantity	Fat	Protein	Carbs	Fibre	kJ/Cal
Breakfast 1 2 3 4 5 ○ ○ ○ ○ ○ HUNGER SCALE								
Mid-morning ○ ○ ○ ○								
Lunch 1 2 3 4 5 ○ ○ ○ ○ ○ HUNGER SCALE								
Mid-afternoon ○ ○ ○ ○								
Dinner 1 2 3 4 5 ○ ○ ○ ○ ○ HUNGER SCALE								
Evening ○ ○ ○ ○								

Coffees/teas　　Fluid intake ▽▽▽▽▽▽▽▽▽▽　Daily totals

TUESDAY

	Time		Quantity	Fat	Protein	Carbs	Fibre	kJ/Cal
Breakfast 1 2 3 4 5 ○ ○ ○ ○ ○ HUNGER SCALE								
Mid-morning ○ ○ ○ ○								
Lunch 1 2 3 4 5 ○ ○ ○ ○ ○ HUNGER SCALE								
Mid-afternoon ○ ○ ○ ○								
Dinner 1 2 3 4 5 ○ ○ ○ ○ ○ HUNGER SCALE								
Evening ○ ○ ○ ○								

Coffees/teas　　Fluid intake ▽▽▽▽▽▽▽▽▽▽　Daily totals

WEDNESDAY

Time

		Quantity	Fat	Protein	Carbs	Fibre	kJ/Cal
Breakfast 1 2 3 4 5 ○ ○ ○ ○ ○ HUNGER SCALE							
Mid-morning ○ ○ ○ ○ ○							
Lunch 1 2 3 4 5 ○ ○ ○ ○ ○ HUNGER SCALE							
Mid-afternoon ○ ○ ○ ○ ○							
Dinner 1 2 3 4 5 ○ ○ ○ ○ ○ HUNGER SCALE							
Evening ○ ○ ○ ○ ○							

Coffees/teas   Fluid intake ☐ ☐ ☐ ☐ ☐ ☐ ☐ ☐ ☐ ☐   Daily totals

THURSDAY

		Quantity	Fat	Protein	Carbs	Fibre	kJ/Cal
Breakfast 1 2 3 4 5 ○ ○ ○ ○ ○ HUNGER SCALE							
Mid-morning ○ ○ ○ ○ ○							
Lunch 1 2 3 4 5 ○ ○ ○ ○ ○ HUNGER SCALE							
Mid-afternoon ○ ○ ○ ○ ○							
Dinner 1 2 3 4 5 ○ ○ ○ ○ ○ HUNGER SCALE							
Evening ○ ○ ○ ○ ○							

Coffees/teas   Fluid intake ☐ ☐ ☐ ☐ ☐ ☐ ☐ ☐ ☐ ☐   Daily totals

FRIDAY

		Quantity	Fat	Protein	Carbs	Fibre	kJ/Cal
Breakfast 1 2 3 4 5 ○ ○ ○ ○ ○ HUNGER SCALE							
Mid-morning ○ ○ ○ ○ ○							
Lunch 1 2 3 4 5 ○ ○ ○ ○ ○ HUNGER SCALE							
Mid-afternoon ○ ○ ○ ○ ○							
Dinner 1 2 3 4 5 ○ ○ ○ ○ ○ HUNGER SCALE							
Evening ○ ○ ○ ○ ○							

Coffees/teas   Fluid intake ☐ ☐ ☐ ☐ ☐ ☐ ☐ ☐ ☐ ☐   Daily totals

SATURDAY

	Time		Quantity	Fat	Protein	Carbs	Fibre	kJ/Cal
Breakfast 1 2 3 4 5 ○ ○ ○ ○ ○ HUNGER SCALE								
Mid-morning ○ ○ ○ ○ ○								
Lunch 1 2 3 4 5 ○ ○ ○ ○ ○ HUNGER SCALE								
Mid-afternoon ○ ○ ○ ○ ○								
Dinner 1 2 3 4 5 ○ ○ ○ ○ ○ HUNGER SCALE								
Evening ○ ○ ○ ○ ○								

Coffees/teas | **Fluid intake** ▽▽▽▽▽▽▽▽▽▽ | **Daily totals**

SUNDAY

	Time		Quantity	Fat	Protein	Carbs	Fibre	kJ/Cal
Breakfast 1 2 3 4 5 ○ ○ ○ ○ ○ HUNGER SCALE								
Mid-morning ○ ○ ○ ○ ○								
Lunch 1 2 3 4 5 ○ ○ ○ ○ ○ HUNGER SCALE								
Mid-afternoon ○ ○ ○ ○ ○								
Dinner 1 2 3 4 5 ○ ○ ○ ○ ○ HUNGER SCALE								
Evening ○ ○ ○ ○ ○								

Coffees/teas | **Fluid intake** ▽▽▽▽▽▽▽▽▽▽ | **Daily totals**

Units of alcohol this week   **Total alcohol kJ/Cal**

Vitamins and supplements

	Fat	Protein	Carbs	Fibre	kJ/Cal
WEEKLY TOTALS					

WEEKLY PERSONAL SUMMARY

Mood 1 2 3 4 5 ○ ○ ○ ○ ○   **Appetite** 1 2 3 4 5 ○ ○ ○ ○ ○

Energy level 1 2 3 4 5 ○ ○ ○ ○ ○   **Stress level** 1 2 3 4 5 ○ ○ ○ ○ ○

Hours of sleep   **Sleep quality** 1 2 3 4 5 ○ ○ ○ ○ ○

kJ/Cal intake

Planned kJ/Cal	
Actual kJ/Cal	
Difference [+/-]	

Weight at end of week

BMI at end of week

Injuries or illnesses

88

EXERCISE DIARY

STRENGTH TRAINING		SET 1		SET 2		SET 3		SET4			
Exercise	Focus area	Reps	Weight	Reps	Weight	Reps	Weight	Reps	Weight	Equipment	Ease

CARDIO TRAINING

Exercise	Time	Distance	Intensity	Heart rate	Ease	kJ/Cal burnt

Total kJ/Cal burnt

INCIDENTAL EXERCISE

Day	Activity	Day	Activity

WEEK BEGINNING   /   /

Weight at start of week

BMI at start of week

Planned kJ/Cal this week

Possible diet-busting occasions this week

Planned exercise sessions this week

	Exercise	Completed [Y/N]
Monday		
Tuesday		
Wednesday		
Thursday		
Friday		
Saturday		
Sunday		

FOOD DIARY

MONDAY

	Time		Quantity	Fat	Protein	Carbs	Fibre	kJ/Cal
Breakfast 1 2 3 4 5 ○○○○○ HUNGER SCALE								
Mid-morning ○○○○○								
Lunch 1 2 3 4 5 ○○○○○ HUNGER SCALE								
Mid-afternoon ○○○○○								
Dinner 1 2 3 4 5 ○○○○○ HUNGER SCALE								
Evening ○○○○○								

Coffees/teas   Fluid intake ▽▽▽▽▽▽▽▽▽▽   Daily totals

TUESDAY

	Time		Quantity	Fat	Protein	Carbs	Fibre	kJ/Cal
Breakfast 1 2 3 4 5 ○○○○○ HUNGER SCALE								
Mid-morning ○○○○○								
Lunch 1 2 3 4 5 ○○○○○ HUNGER SCALE								
Mid-afternoon ○○○○○								
Dinner 1 2 3 4 5 ○○○○○ HUNGER SCALE								
Evening ○○○○○								

Coffees/teas   Fluid intake ▽▽▽▽▽▽▽▽▽▽   Daily totals

WEDNESDAY

	Time		Quantity	Fat	Protein	Carbs	Fibre	kJ/Cal
Breakfast 1 2 3 4 5 ○○○○○ HUNGER SCALE								
Mid-morning ○○○○○								
Lunch 1 2 3 4 5 ○○○○○ HUNGER SCALE								
Mid-afternoon ○○○○○								
Dinner 1 2 3 4 5 ○○○○○ HUNGER SCALE								
Evening ○○○○○								

Coffees/teas   Fluid intake ⊔⊔⊔⊔⊔⊔⊔⊔⊔⊔   Daily totals

THURSDAY

	Time		Quantity	Fat	Protein	Carbs	Fibre	kJ/Cal
Breakfast 1 2 3 4 5 ○○○○○ HUNGER SCALE								
Mid-morning ○○○○○								
Lunch 1 2 3 4 5 ○○○○○ HUNGER SCALE								
Mid-afternoon ○○○○○								
Dinner 1 2 3 4 5 ○○○○○ HUNGER SCALE								
Evening ○○○○○								

Coffees/teas   Fluid intake ⊔⊔⊔⊔⊔⊔⊔⊔⊔⊔   Daily totals

FRIDAY

	Time		Quantity	Fat	Protein	Carbs	Fibre	kJ/Cal
Breakfast 1 2 3 4 5 ○○○○○ HUNGER SCALE								
Mid-morning ○○○○○								
Lunch 1 2 3 4 5 ○○○○○ HUNGER SCALE								
Mid-afternoon ○○○○○								
Dinner 1 2 3 4 5 ○○○○○ HUNGER SCALE								
Evening ○○○○○								

Coffees/teas   Fluid intake ⊔⊔⊔⊔⊔⊔⊔⊔⊔⊔   Daily totals

SATURDAY

	Time						Quantity	Fat	Protein	Carbs	Fibre	kJ/Cal
Breakfast 1 2 3 4 5 ○○○○○ HUNGER SCALE												
Mid-morning ○○○○○												
Lunch 1 2 3 4 5 ○○○○○ HUNGER SCALE												
Mid-afternoon ○○○○○												
Dinner 1 2 3 4 5 ○○○○○ HUNGER SCALE												
Evening ○○○○○												

Coffees/teas   Fluid intake 🥛🥛🥛🥛🥛🥛🥛🥛🥛🥛   Daily totals

SUNDAY

	Time						Quantity	Fat	Protein	Carbs	Fibre	kJ/Cal
Breakfast 1 2 3 4 5 ○○○○○ HUNGER SCALE												
Mid-morning ○○○○○												
Lunch 1 2 3 4 5 ○○○○○ HUNGER SCALE												
Mid-afternoon ○○○○○												
Dinner 1 2 3 4 5 ○○○○○ HUNGER SCALE												
Evening ○○○○○												

Coffees/teas   Fluid intake 🥛🥛🥛🥛🥛🥛🥛🥛🥛🥛   Daily totals

Units of alcohol this week   Total alcohol kJ/Cal

Vitamins and supplements

	Fat	Protein	Carbs	Fibre	kJ/Cal
WEEKLY TOTALS					

WEEKLY PERSONAL SUMMARY

Mood 1 2 3 4 5 ○○○○○   **Appetite** 1 2 3 4 5 ○○○○○

Energy level 1 2 3 4 5 ○○○○○   **Stress level** 1 2 3 4 5 ○○○○○

Hours of sleep   **Sleep quality** 1 2 3 4 5 ○○○○○

Injuries or illnesses

kJ/Cal intake	
Planned kJ/Cal	
Actual kJ/Cal	
Difference [+/-]	

Weight at end of week

BMI at end of week

EXERCISE DIARY

STRENGTH TRAINING		SET 1		SET 2		SET 3		SET4			
Exercise	Focus area	Reps	Weight	Reps	Weight	Reps	Weight	Reps	Weight	Equipment	Ease

CARDIO TRAINING

Exercise	Time	Distance	Intensity	Heart rate	Ease	kJ/Cal burnt

Total kJ/Cal burnt

INCIDENTAL EXERCISE

Day	Activity	Day	Activity

WEEK BEGINNING   /   /

Weight at start of week

BMI at start of week

Planned kJ/Cal this week

Possible diet-busting occasions this week

Planned exercise sessions this week

	Exercise	Completed [Y/N]
Monday		
Tuesday		
Wednesday		
Thursday		
Friday		
Saturday		
Sunday		

FOOD DIARY

MONDAY

Time		Quantity	Fat	Protein	Carbs	Fibre	kJ/Cal
Breakfast 1 2 3 4 5 ○ ○ ○ ○ ○ HUNGER SCALE							
Mid-morning ○ ○ ○ ○ ○							
Lunch 1 2 3 4 5 ○ ○ ○ ○ ○ HUNGER SCALE							
Mid-afternoon ○ ○ ○ ○ ○							
Dinner 1 2 3 4 5 ○ ○ ○ ○ ○ HUNGER SCALE							
Evening ○ ○ ○ ○ ○							

Coffees/teas   Fluid intake 🥛🥛🥛🥛🥛🥛🥛🥛🥛🥛   Daily totals

TUESDAY

		Quantity	Fat	Protein	Carbs	Fibre	kJ/Cal
Breakfast 1 2 3 4 5 ○ ○ ○ ○ ○ HUNGER SCALE							
Mid-morning ○ ○ ○ ○ ○							
Lunch 1 2 3 4 5 ○ ○ ○ ○ ○ HUNGER SCALE							
Mid-afternoon ○ ○ ○ ○ ○							
Dinner 1 2 3 4 5 ○ ○ ○ ○ ○ HUNGER SCALE							
Evening ○ ○ ○ ○ ○							

Coffees/teas   Fluid intake 🥛🥛🥛🥛🥛🥛🥛🥛🥛🥛   Daily totals

WEDNESDAY

	Time		Quantity	Fat	Protein	Carbs	Fibre	kJ/Cal
Breakfast 1 2 3 4 5 ○○○○○ HUNGER SCALE								
Mid-morning ○○○○○								
Lunch 1 2 3 4 5 ○○○○○ HUNGER SCALE								
Mid-afternoon ○○○○○								
Dinner 1 2 3 4 5 ○○○○○ HUNGER SCALE								
Evening ○○○○○								

Coffees/teas ▢ Fluid intake ⊔⊔⊔⊔⊔⊔⊔⊔⊔⊔ Daily totals

THURSDAY

	Time		Quantity	Fat	Protein	Carbs	Fibre	kJ/Cal
Breakfast 1 2 3 4 5 ○○○○○ HUNGER SCALE								
Mid-morning ○○○○○								
Lunch 1 2 3 4 5 ○○○○○ HUNGER SCALE								
Mid-afternoon ○○○○○								
Dinner 1 2 3 4 5 ○○○○○ HUNGER SCALE								
Evening ○○○○○								

Coffees/teas ▢ Fluid intake ⊔⊔⊔⊔⊔⊔⊔⊔⊔⊔ Daily totals

FRIDAY

	Time		Quantity	Fat	Protein	Carbs	Fibre	kJ/Cal
Breakfast 1 2 3 4 5 ○○○○○ HUNGER SCALE								
Mid-morning ○○○○○								
Lunch 1 2 3 4 5 ○○○○○ HUNGER SCALE								
Mid-afternoon ○○○○○								
Dinner 1 2 3 4 5 ○○○○○ HUNGER SCALE								
Evening ○○○○○								

Coffees/teas ▢ Fluid intake ⊔⊔⊔⊔⊔⊔⊔⊔⊔⊔ Daily totals

SATURDAY

	Time				Quantity	Fat	Protein	Carbs	Fibre	kJ/Cal
Breakfast 1 2 3 4 5 ○ ○ ○ ○ ○ HUNGER SCALE										
Mid-morning ○ ○ ○ ○ ○										
Lunch 1 2 3 4 5 ○ ○ ○ ○ ○ HUNGER SCALE										
Mid-afternoon ○ ○ ○ ○ ○										
Dinner 1 2 3 4 5 ○ ○ ○ ○ ○ HUNGER SCALE										
Evening ○ ○ ○ ○ ○										

Coffees/teas   Fluid intake ⛀⛀⛀⛀⛀⛀⛀⛀⛀⛀   Daily totals

SUNDAY

	Time				Quantity	Fat	Protein	Carbs	Fibre	kJ/Cal
Breakfast 1 2 3 4 5 ○ ○ ○ ○ ○ HUNGER SCALE										
Mid-morning ○ ○ ○ ○ ○										
Lunch 1 2 3 4 5 ○ ○ ○ ○ ○ HUNGER SCALE										
Mid-afternoon ○ ○ ○ ○ ○										
Dinner 1 2 3 4 5 ○ ○ ○ ○ ○ HUNGER SCALE										
Evening ○ ○ ○ ○ ○										

Coffees/teas   Fluid intake ⛀⛀⛀⛀⛀⛀⛀⛀⛀⛀   Daily totals

Units of alcohol this week   **Total alcohol kJ/Cal**

Vitamins and supplements

WEEKLY TOTALS	Fat	Protein	Carbs	Fibre	kJ/Cal

WEEKLY PERSONAL SUMMARY

Mood 1 2 3 4 5 ○ ○ ○ ○ ○   **Appetite** 1 2 3 4 5 ○ ○ ○ ○ ○

Energy level 1 2 3 4 5 ○ ○ ○ ○ ○   **Stress level** 1 2 3 4 5 ○ ○ ○ ○ ○

Hours of sleep [ ]   **Sleep quality** 1 2 3 4 5 ○ ○ ○ ○ ○

kJ/Cal intake

Planned kJ/Cal	
Actual kJ/Cal	

Difference [+/-]

Weight at end of week

BMI at end of week

Injuries or illnesses

EXERCISE DIARY

STRENGTH TRAINING		SET 1		SET 2		SET 3		SET 4			
Exercise	Focus area	Reps	Weight	Reps	Weight	Reps	Weight	Reps	Weight	Equipment	Ease

CARDIO TRAINING

Exercise	Time	Distance	Intensity	Heart rate	Ease	kJ/Cal burnt

Total kJ/Cal burnt

INCIDENTAL EXERCISE

Day	Activity	Day	Activity

WEEK BEGINNING   /   /

Weight at start of week   ▭

BMI at start of week   ▭

Planned kJ/Cal this week   ▭

Possible diet-busting occasions this week

Planned exercise sessions this week

	Exercise	Completed [Y/N]
Monday		
Tuesday		
Wednesday		
Thursday		
Friday		
Saturday		
Sunday		

FOOD DIARY

MONDAY

	Time		Quantity	Fat	Protein	Carbs	Fibre	kJ/Cal
Breakfast 1 2 3 4 5 ○ ○ ○ ○ ○ HUNGER SCALE								
Mid-morning ○ ○ ○ ○ ○								
Lunch 1 2 3 4 5 ○ ○ ○ ○ ○ HUNGER SCALE								
Mid-afternoon ○ ○ ○ ○ ○								
Dinner 1 2 3 4 5 ○ ○ ○ ○ ○ HUNGER SCALE								
Evening ○ ○ ○ ○ ○								

Coffees/teas ▭   Fluid intake 🥤🥤🥤🥤🥤🥤🥤🥤🥤   Daily totals

TUESDAY

	Time		Quantity	Fat	Protein	Carbs	Fibre	kJ/Cal
Breakfast 1 2 3 4 5 ○ ○ ○ ○ ○ HUNGER SCALE								
Mid-morning ○ ○ ○ ○ ○								
Lunch 1 2 3 4 5 ○ ○ ○ ○ ○ HUNGER SCALE								
Mid-afternoon ○ ○ ○ ○ ○								
Dinner 1 2 3 4 5 ○ ○ ○ ○ ○ HUNGER SCALE								
Evening ○ ○ ○ ○ ○								

Coffees/teas ▭   Fluid intake 🥤🥤🥤🥤🥤🥤🥤🥤🥤   Daily totals

WEDNESDAY

	Time		Quantity	Fat	Protein	Carbs	Fibre	kJ/Cal
Breakfast 1 2 3 4 5 ○○○○○ HUNGER SCALE								
Mid-morning ○○○○○								
Lunch 1 2 3 4 5 ○○○○○ HUNGER SCALE								
Mid-afternoon ○○○○○								
Dinner 1 2 3 4 5 ○○○○○ HUNGER SCALE								
Evening ○○○○○								

Coffees/teas ___ Fluid intake ⛆⛆⛆⛆⛆⛆⛆⛆⛆⛆ Daily totals

THURSDAY

	Time		Quantity	Fat	Protein	Carbs	Fibre	kJ/Cal
Breakfast 1 2 3 4 5 ○○○○○ HUNGER SCALE								
Mid-morning ○○○○○								
Lunch 1 2 3 4 5 ○○○○○ HUNGER SCALE								
Mid-afternoon ○○○○○								
Dinner 1 2 3 4 5 ○○○○○ HUNGER SCALE								
Evening ○○○○○								

Coffees/teas ___ Fluid intake ⛆⛆⛆⛆⛆⛆⛆⛆⛆⛆ Daily totals

FRIDAY

	Time		Quantity	Fat	Protein	Carbs	Fibre	kJ/Cal
Breakfast 1 2 3 4 5 ○○○○○ HUNGER SCALE								
Mid-morning ○○○○○								
Lunch 1 2 3 4 5 ○○○○○ HUNGER SCALE								
Mid-afternoon ○○○○○								
Dinner 1 2 3 4 5 ○○○○○ HUNGER SCALE								
Evening ○○○○○								

Coffees/teas ___ Fluid intake ⛆⛆⛆⛆⛆⛆⛆⛆⛆⛆ Daily totals

SATURDAY

	Time		Quantity	Fat	Protein	Carbs	Fibre	kJ/Cal
Breakfast 1 2 3 4 5 ○○○○○ HUNGER SCALE								
Mid-morning ○○○○○								
Lunch 1 2 3 4 5 ○○○○○ HUNGER SCALE								
Mid-afternoon ○○○○○								
Dinner 1 2 3 4 5 ○○○○○ HUNGER SCALE								
Evening ○○○○○								

Coffees/teas ☐ Fluid intake ⊔⊔⊔⊔⊔⊔⊔⊔⊔⊔ Daily totals

SUNDAY

	Time		Quantity	Fat	Protein	Carbs	Fibre	kJ/Cal
Breakfast 1 2 3 4 5 ○○○○○ HUNGER SCALE								
Mid-morning ○○○○○								
Lunch 1 2 3 4 5 ○○○○○ HUNGER SCALE								
Mid-afternoon ○○○○○								
Dinner 1 2 3 4 5 ○○○○○ HUNGER SCALE								
Evening ○○○○○								

Coffees/teas ☐ Fluid intake ⊔⊔⊔⊔⊔⊔⊔⊔⊔⊔ Daily totals

Units of alcohol this week ☐   Total alcohol kJ/Cal ☐

Vitamins and supplements

WEEKLY TOTALS	Fat	Protein	Carbs	Fibre	kJ/Cal

WEEKLY PERSONAL SUMMARY

Mood 1 2 3 4 5 ○○○○○ **Appetite** 1 2 3 4 5 ○○○○○

Energy level 1 2 3 4 5 ○○○○○ **Stress level** 1 2 3 4 5 ○○○○○

Hours of sleep ☐ **Sleep quality** 1 2 3 4 5 ○○○○○

Injuries or illnesses

kJ/Cal intake

Planned kJ/Cal	
Actual kJ/Cal	
Difference [+/-]	

Weight at end of week ☐

BMI at end of week ☐

EXERCISE DIARY

STRENGTH TRAINING

Exercise	Focus area	SET 1		SET 2		SET 3		SET4		Equipment	Ease
		Reps	Weight	Reps	Weight	Reps	Weight	Reps	Weight		

CARDIO TRAINING

Exercise	Time	Distance	Intensity	Heart rate	Ease	kJ/Cal burnt

Total kJ/Cal burnt

INCIDENTAL EXERCISE

Day	Activity	Day	Activity

WEEK BEGINNING   /   /

Weight at start of week

BMI at start of week

Planned kJ/Cal this week

Possible diet-busting occasions this week

Planned exercise sessions this week

	Exercise	Completed [Y/N]
Monday		
Tuesday		
Wednesday		
Thursday		
Friday		
Saturday		
Sunday		

FOOD DIARY

MONDAY

	Time		Quantity	Fat	Protein	Carbs	Fibre	kJ/Cal
Breakfast 1 2 3 4 5 ○ ○ ○ ○ ○ HUNGER SCALE								
Mid-morning ○ ○ ○ ○ ○								
Lunch 1 2 3 4 5 ○ ○ ○ ○ ○ HUNGER SCALE								
Mid-afternoon ○ ○ ○ ○ ○								
Dinner 1 2 3 4 5 ○ ○ ○ ○ ○ HUNGER SCALE								
Evening ○ ○ ○ ○ ○								

Coffees/teas   Fluid intake ⛀ ⛀ ⛀ ⛀ ⛀ ⛀ ⛀ ⛀ ⛀ ⛀   Daily totals

TUESDAY

	Time		Quantity	Fat	Protein	Carbs	Fibre	kJ/Cal
Breakfast 1 2 3 4 5 ○ ○ ○ ○ ○ HUNGER SCALE								
Mid-morning ○ ○ ○ ○ ○								
Lunch 1 2 3 4 5 ○ ○ ○ ○ ○ HUNGER SCALE								
Mid-afternoon ○ ○ ○ ○ ○								
Dinner 1 2 3 4 5 ○ ○ ○ ○ ○ HUNGER SCALE								
Evening ○ ○ ○ ○ ○								

Coffees/teas   Fluid intake ⛀ ⛀ ⛀ ⛀ ⛀ ⛀ ⛀ ⛀ ⛀ ⛀   Daily totals

WEDNESDAY

	Time		Quantity	Fat	Protein	Carbs	Fibre	kJ/Cal
Breakfast 1 2 3 4 5 ○ ○ ○ ○ ○ HUNGER SCALE								
Mid-morning ○ ○ ○ ○ ○								
Lunch 1 2 3 4 5 ○ ○ ○ ○ ○ HUNGER SCALE								
Mid-afternoon ○ ○ ○ ○ ○								
Dinner 1 2 3 4 5 ○ ○ ○ ○ ○ HUNGER SCALE								
Evening ○ ○ ○ ○ ○								

Coffees/teas   Fluid intake ▽▽▽▽▽▽▽▽▽▽   Daily totals

THURSDAY

	Time		Quantity	Fat	Protein	Carbs	Fibre	kJ/Cal
Breakfast 1 2 3 4 5 ○ ○ ○ ○ ○ HUNGER SCALE								
Mid-morning ○ ○ ○ ○ ○								
Lunch 1 2 3 4 5 ○ ○ ○ ○ ○ HUNGER SCALE								
Mid-afternoon ○ ○ ○ ○ ○								
Dinner 1 2 3 4 5 ○ ○ ○ ○ ○ HUNGER SCALE								
Evening ○ ○ ○ ○ ○								

Coffees/teas   Fluid intake ▽▽▽▽▽▽▽▽▽▽   Daily totals

FRIDAY

	Time		Quantity	Fat	Protein	Carbs	Fibre	kJ/Cal
Breakfast 1 2 3 4 5 ○ ○ ○ ○ ○ HUNGER SCALE								
Mid-morning ○ ○ ○ ○ ○								
Lunch 1 2 3 4 5 ○ ○ ○ ○ ○ HUNGER SCALE								
Mid-afternoon ○ ○ ○ ○ ○								
Dinner 1 2 3 4 5 ○ ○ ○ ○ ○ HUNGER SCALE								
Evening ○ ○ ○ ○ ○								

Coffees/teas   Fluid intake ▽▽▽▽▽▽▽▽▽▽   Daily totals

SATURDAY

	Time		Quantity	Fat	Protein	Carbs	Fibre	kJ/Cal
Breakfast 1 2 3 4 5 ○ ○ ○ ○ ○ HUNGER SCALE								
Mid-morning ○ ○ ○ ○ ○								
Lunch 1 2 3 4 5 ○ ○ ○ ○ ○ HUNGER SCALE								
Mid-afternoon ○ ○ ○ ○ ○								
Dinner 1 2 3 4 5 ○ ○ ○ ○ ○ HUNGER SCALE								
Evening ○ ○ ○ ○ ○								

Coffees/teas ☐   Fluid intake ⊔ ⊔ ⊔ ⊔ ⊔ ⊔ ⊔ ⊔ ⊔ ⊔   Daily totals

SUNDAY

	Time		Quantity	Fat	Protein	Carbs	Fibre	kJ/Cal
Breakfast 1 2 3 4 5 ○ ○ ○ ○ ○ HUNGER SCALE								
Mid-morning ○ ○ ○ ○ ○								
Lunch 1 2 3 4 5 ○ ○ ○ ○ ○ HUNGER SCALE								
Mid-afternoon ○ ○ ○ ○ ○								
Dinner 1 2 3 4 5 ○ ○ ○ ○ ○ HUNGER SCALE								
Evening ○ ○ ○ ○ ○								

Coffees/teas ☐   Fluid intake ⊔ ⊔ ⊔ ⊔ ⊔ ⊔ ⊔ ⊔ ⊔ ⊔   Daily totals

Units of alcohol this week ☐   **Total alcohol kJ/Cal**

Vitamins and supplements

WEEKLY TOTALS	Fat	Protein	Carbs	Fibre	kJ/Cal

WEEKLY PERSONAL SUMMARY

Mood 1 2 3 4 5 ○ ○ ○ ○ ○   **Appetite** 1 2 3 4 5 ○ ○ ○ ○ ○

Energy level 1 2 3 4 5 ○ ○ ○ ○ ○   **Stress level** 1 2 3 4 5 ○ ○ ○ ○ ○

Hours of sleep ☐   **Sleep quality** 1 2 3 4 5 ○ ○ ○ ○ ○

Injuries or illnesses

kJ/Cal intake

Planned kJ/Cal	
Actual kJ/Cal	

Difference [+/-]

Weight at end of week

BMI at end of week

EXERCISE DIARY

STRENGTH TRAINING		SET 1		SET 2		SET 3		SET4			
Exercise	Focus area	Reps	Weight	Reps	Weight	Reps	Weight	Reps	Weight	Equipment	Ease

CARDIO TRAINING

Exercise	Time	Distance	Intensity	Heart rate	Ease	kJ/Cal burnt

Total kJ/Cal burnt

INCIDENTAL EXERCISE

Day	Activity	Day	Activity

WEEK BEGINNING ___/___/___

Weight at start of week _____

BMI at start of week _____

Planned kJ/Cal this week _____

Possible diet-busting occasions this week

Planned exercise sessions this week

	Exercise	Completed [Y/N]
Monday		
Tuesday		
Wednesday		
Thursday		
Friday		
Saturday		
Sunday		

FOOD DIARY

MONDAY

Time		Quantity	Fat	Protein	Carbs	Fibre	kJ/Cal
Breakfast 1 2 3 4 5 ○○○○○ HUNGER SCALE							
Mid-morning ○○○○○							
Lunch 1 2 3 4 5 ○○○○○ HUNGER SCALE							
Mid-afternoon ○○○○○							
Dinner 1 2 3 4 5 ○○○○○ HUNGER SCALE							
Evening ○○○○○							

Coffees/teas _____   Fluid intake ⊔⊔⊔⊔⊔⊔⊔⊔⊔⊔   Daily totals

TUESDAY

Time		Quantity	Fat	Protein	Carbs	Fibre	kJ/Cal
Breakfast 1 2 3 4 5 ○○○○○ HUNGER SCALE							
Mid-morning ○○○○○							
Lunch 1 2 3 4 5 ○○○○○ HUNGER SCALE							
Mid-afternoon ○○○○○							
Dinner 1 2 3 4 5 ○○○○○ HUNGER SCALE							
Evening ○○○○○							

Coffees/teas _____   Fluid intake ⊔⊔⊔⊔⊔⊔⊔⊔⊔⊔   Daily totals

WEDNESDAY

	Time		Quantity	Fat	Protein	Carbs	Fibre	kJ/Cal
Breakfast								
1 2 3 4 5 ○○○○○ HUNGER SCALE								
Mid-morning ○○○○○								
Lunch								
1 2 3 4 5 ○○○○○ HUNGER SCALE								
Mid-afternoon ○○○○○								
Dinner								
1 2 3 4 5 ○○○○○ HUNGER SCALE								
Evening ○○○○○								
Coffees/teas		Fluid intake ▽▽▽▽▽▽▽▽▽▽	Daily totals					

THURSDAY

	Time		Quantity	Fat	Protein	Carbs	Fibre	kJ/Cal
Breakfast								
1 2 3 4 5 ○○○○○ HUNGER SCALE								
Mid-morning ○○○○○								
Lunch								
1 2 3 4 5 ○○○○○ HUNGER SCALE								
Mid-afternoon ○○○○○								
Dinner								
1 2 3 4 5 ○○○○○ HUNGER SCALE								
Evening ○○○○○								
Coffees/teas		Fluid intake ▽▽▽▽▽▽▽▽▽▽	Daily totals					

FRIDAY

	Time		Quantity	Fat	Protein	Carbs	Fibre	kJ/Cal
Breakfast								
1 2 3 4 5 ○○○○○ HUNGER SCALE								
Mid-morning ○○○○○								
Lunch								
1 2 3 4 5 ○○○○○ HUNGER SCALE								
Mid-afternoon ○○○○○								
Dinner								
1 2 3 4 5 ○○○○○ HUNGER SCALE								
Evening ○○○○○								
Coffees/teas		Fluid intake ▽▽▽▽▽▽▽▽▽▽	Daily totals					

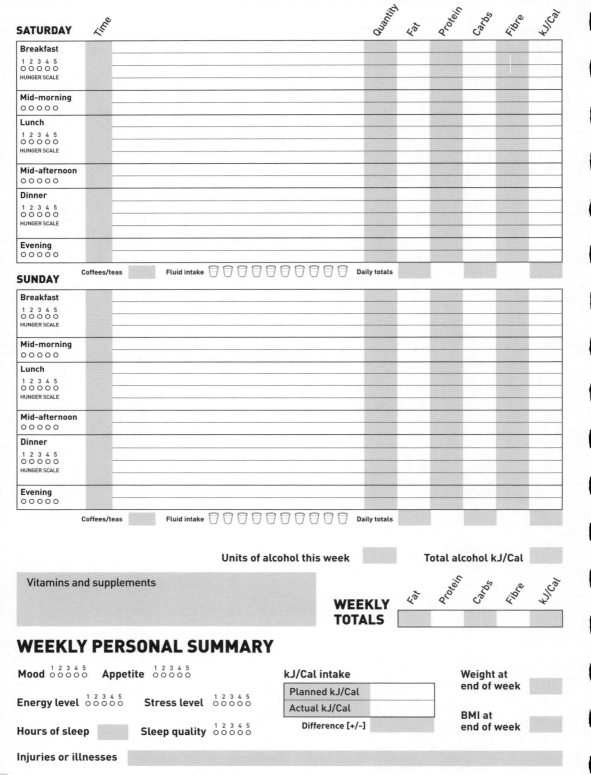

SATURDAY

	Time								Quantity	Fat	Protein	Carbs	Fibre	kJ/Cal
Breakfast 1 2 3 4 5 ○○○○○ HUNGER SCALE														
Mid-morning ○○○○○														
Lunch 1 2 3 4 5 ○○○○○ HUNGER SCALE														
Mid-afternoon ○○○○○														
Dinner 1 2 3 4 5 ○○○○○ HUNGER SCALE														
Evening ○○○○○														
Coffees/teas	Fluid intake 🥤🥤🥤🥤🥤🥤🥤🥤🥤🥤								Daily totals					

SUNDAY

	Time								Quantity	Fat	Protein	Carbs	Fibre	kJ/Cal
Breakfast 1 2 3 4 5 ○○○○○ HUNGER SCALE														
Mid-morning ○○○○○														
Lunch 1 2 3 4 5 ○○○○○ HUNGER SCALE														
Mid-afternoon ○○○○○														
Dinner 1 2 3 4 5 ○○○○○ HUNGER SCALE														
Evening ○○○○○														
Coffees/teas	Fluid intake 🥤🥤🥤🥤🥤🥤🥤🥤🥤🥤								Daily totals					

Units of alcohol this week   **Total alcohol kJ/Cal**

Vitamins and supplements

	Fat	Protein	Carbs	Fibre	kJ/Cal
WEEKLY TOTALS					

WEEKLY PERSONAL SUMMARY

Mood 1 2 3 4 5 ○○○○○   **Appetite** 1 2 3 4 5 ○○○○○

Energy level 1 2 3 4 5 ○○○○○   **Stress level** 1 2 3 4 5 ○○○○○

Hours of sleep   **Sleep quality** 1 2 3 4 5 ○○○○○

kJ/Cal intake

Planned kJ/Cal	
Actual kJ/Cal	
Difference [+/-]	

Weight at end of week

BMI at end of week

Injuries or illnesses

EXERCISE DIARY

STRENGTH TRAINING		SET 1		SET 2		SET 3		SET 4			
Exercise	Focus area	Reps	Weight	Reps	Weight	Reps	Weight	Reps	Weight	Equipment	Ease

CARDIO TRAINING

Exercise	Time	Distance	Intensity	Heart rate	Ease	kJ/Cal burnt

Total kJ/Cal burnt

INCIDENTAL EXERCISE

Day	Activity	Day	Activity

WEEK BEGINNING   /   /

Weight at start of week

BMI at start of week

Planned kJ/Cal this week

Possible diet-busting occasions this week

Planned exercise sessions this week

	Exercise	Completed [Y/N]
Monday		
Tuesday		
Wednesday		
Thursday		
Friday		
Saturday		
Sunday		

FOOD DIARY

MONDAY

	Time		Quantity	Fat	Protein	Carbs	Fibre	kJ/Cal
Breakfast 1 2 3 4 5 ○ ○ ○ ○ ○ HUNGER SCALE								
Mid-morning ○ ○ ○ ○ ○								
Lunch 1 2 3 4 5 ○ ○ ○ ○ ○ HUNGER SCALE								
Mid-afternoon ○ ○ ○ ○ ○								
Dinner 1 2 3 4 5 ○ ○ ○ ○ ○ HUNGER SCALE								
Evening ○ ○ ○ ○ ○								

Coffees/teas ☐   Fluid intake ▽▽▽▽▽▽▽▽▽▽   Daily totals

TUESDAY

	Time		Quantity	Fat	Protein	Carbs	Fibre	kJ/Cal
Breakfast 1 2 3 4 5 ○ ○ ○ ○ ○ HUNGER SCALE								
Mid-morning ○ ○ ○ ○ ○								
Lunch 1 2 3 4 5 ○ ○ ○ ○ ○ HUNGER SCALE								
Mid-afternoon ○ ○ ○ ○ ○								
Dinner 1 2 3 4 5 ○ ○ ○ ○ ○ HUNGER SCALE								
Evening ○ ○ ○ ○ ○								

Coffees/teas ☐   Fluid intake ▽▽▽▽▽▽▽▽▽▽   Daily totals

WEDNESDAY

	Time		Quantity	Fat	Protein	Carbs	Fibre	kJ/Cal
Breakfast								
1 2 3 4 5 ○○○○○ HUNGER SCALE								
Mid-morning ○○○○○								
Lunch 1 2 3 4 5 ○○○○○ HUNGER SCALE								
Mid-afternoon ○○○○○								
Dinner 1 2 3 4 5 ○○○○○ HUNGER SCALE								
Evening ○○○○○								

Coffees/teas   Fluid intake ⊔⊔⊔⊔⊔⊔⊔⊔⊔⊔   Daily totals

THURSDAY

Breakfast 1 2 3 4 5 ○○○○○ HUNGER SCALE								
Mid-morning ○○○○○								
Lunch 1 2 3 4 5 ○○○○○ HUNGER SCALE								
Mid-afternoon ○○○○○								
Dinner 1 2 3 4 5 ○○○○○ HUNGER SCALE								
Evening ○○○○○								

Coffees/teas   Fluid intake ⊔⊔⊔⊔⊔⊔⊔⊔⊔⊔   Daily totals

FRIDAY

Breakfast 1 2 3 4 5 ○○○○○ HUNGER SCALE								
Mid-morning ○○○○○								
Lunch 1 2 3 4 5 ○○○○○ HUNGER SCALE								
Mid-afternoon ○○○○○								
Dinner 1 2 3 4 5 ○○○○○ HUNGER SCALE								
Evening ○○○○○								

Coffees/teas   Fluid intake ⊔⊔⊔⊔⊔⊔⊔⊔⊔⊔   Daily totals

SATURDAY

	Time		Quantity	Fat	Protein	Carbs	Fibre	kJ/Cal
Breakfast 1 2 3 4 5 ○○○○○ HUNGER SCALE								
Mid-morning ○○○○○								
Lunch 1 2 3 4 5 ○○○○○ HUNGER SCALE								
Mid-afternoon ○○○○○								
Dinner 1 2 3 4 5 ○○○○○ HUNGER SCALE								
Evening ○○○○○								

Coffees/teas ▢   Fluid intake ⊔⊔⊔⊔⊔⊔⊔⊔⊔⊔   Daily totals

SUNDAY

	Time		Quantity	Fat	Protein	Carbs	Fibre	kJ/Cal
Breakfast 1 2 3 4 5 ○○○○○ HUNGER SCALE								
Mid-morning ○○○○○								
Lunch 1 2 3 4 5 ○○○○○ HUNGER SCALE								
Mid-afternoon ○○○○○								
Dinner 1 2 3 4 5 ○○○○○ HUNGER SCALE								
Evening ○○○○○								

Coffees/teas ▢   Fluid intake ⊔⊔⊔⊔⊔⊔⊔⊔⊔⊔   Daily totals

Units of alcohol this week ▢   Total alcohol kJ/Cal ▢

Vitamins and supplements

	Fat	Protein	Carbs	Fibre	kJ/Cal
WEEKLY TOTALS					

WEEKLY PERSONAL SUMMARY

Mood 1 2 3 4 5 ○○○○○   **Appetite** 1 2 3 4 5 ○○○○○

Energy level 1 2 3 4 5 ○○○○○   **Stress level** 1 2 3 4 5 ○○○○○

Hours of sleep ▢   **Sleep quality** 1 2 3 4 5 ○○○○○

Injuries or illnesses

kJ/Cal intake

Planned kJ/Cal	
Actual kJ/Cal	
Difference [+/-]	

Weight at end of week

BMI at end of week

EXERCISE DIARY

STRENGTH TRAINING

Exercise	Focus area	SET 1 Reps	SET 1 Weight	SET 2 Reps	SET 2 Weight	SET 3 Reps	SET 3 Weight	SET4 Reps	SET4 Weight	Equipment	Ease

CARDIO TRAINING

Exercise	Time	Distance	Intensity	Heart rate	Ease	kJ/Cal burnt

Total kJ/Cal burnt

INCIDENTAL EXERCISE

Day	Activity	Day	Activity

WEEK BEGINNING   /   /

Weight at start of week

BMI at start of week

Planned kJ/Cal this week

Possible diet-busting occasions this week

Planned exercise sessions this week

	Exercise	Completed [Y/N]
Monday		
Tuesday		
Wednesday		
Thursday		
Friday		
Saturday		
Sunday		

FOOD DIARY

MONDAY

Time		Quantity	Fat	Protein	Carbs	Fibre	kJ/Cal
Breakfast 1 2 3 4 5 ○○○○○ HUNGER SCALE							
Mid-morning ○○○○○							
Lunch 1 2 3 4 5 ○○○○○ HUNGER SCALE							
Mid-afternoon ○○○○○							
Dinner 1 2 3 4 5 ○○○○○ HUNGER SCALE							
Evening ○○○○							

Coffees/teas   Fluid intake ▽▽▽▽▽▽▽▽▽▽   Daily totals

TUESDAY

Time		Quantity	Fat	Protein	Carbs	Fibre	kJ/Cal
Breakfast 1 2 3 4 5 ○○○○○ HUNGER SCALE							
Mid-morning ○○○○○							
Lunch 1 2 3 4 5 ○○○○○ HUNGER SCALE							
Mid-afternoon ○○○○○							
Dinner 1 2 3 4 5 ○○○○○ HUNGER SCALE							
Evening ○○○○○							

Coffees/teas   Fluid intake ▽▽▽▽▽▽▽▽▽▽   Daily totals

WEDNESDAY

	Time		Quantity	Fat	Protein	Carbs	Fibre	kJ/Cal
Breakfast 1 2 3 4 5 ○○○○○ HUNGER SCALE								
Mid-morning ○○○○○								
Lunch 1 2 3 4 5 ○○○○○ HUNGER SCALE								
Mid-afternoon ○○○○○								
Dinner 1 2 3 4 5 ○○○○○ HUNGER SCALE								
Evening ○○○○○								

Coffees/teas   Fluid intake ▽▽▽▽▽▽▽▽▽▽   Daily totals

THURSDAY

	Time		Quantity	Fat	Protein	Carbs	Fibre	kJ/Cal
Breakfast 1 2 3 4 5 ○○○○○ HUNGER SCALE								
Mid-morning ○○○○○								
Lunch 1 2 3 4 5 ○○○○○ HUNGER SCALE								
Mid-afternoon ○○○○○								
Dinner 1 2 3 4 5 ○○○○○ HUNGER SCALE								
Evening ○○○○○								

Coffees/teas   Fluid intake ▽▽▽▽▽▽▽▽▽▽   Daily totals

FRIDAY

	Time		Quantity	Fat	Protein	Carbs	Fibre	kJ/Cal
Breakfast 1 2 3 4 5 ○○○○○ HUNGER SCALE								
Mid-morning ○○○○○								
Lunch 1 2 3 4 5 ○○○○○ HUNGER SCALE								
Mid-afternoon ○○○○○								
Dinner 1 2 3 4 5 ○○○○○ HUNGER SCALE								
Evening ○○○○○								

Coffees/teas   Fluid intake ▽▽▽▽▽▽▽▽▽▽   Daily totals

SATURDAY

	Time		Quantity	Fat	Protein	Carbs	Fibre	kJ/Cal
Breakfast 1 2 3 4 5 ○○○○○ HUNGER SCALE								
Mid-morning ○○○○○								
Lunch 1 2 3 4 5 ○○○○○ HUNGER SCALE								
Mid-afternoon ○○○○○								
Dinner 1 2 3 4 5 ○○○○○ HUNGER SCALE								
Evening ○○○○○								

Coffees/teas [ ]   Fluid intake ▽▽▽▽▽▽▽▽▽▽   Daily totals

SUNDAY

	Time		Quantity	Fat	Protein	Carbs	Fibre	kJ/Cal
Breakfast 1 2 3 4 5 ○○○○○ HUNGER SCALE								
Mid-morning ○○○○○								
Lunch 1 2 3 4 5 ○○○○○ HUNGER SCALE								
Mid-afternoon ○○○○○								
Dinner 1 2 3 4 5 ○○○○○ HUNGER SCALE								
Evening ○○○○○								

Coffees/teas [ ]   Fluid intake ▽▽▽▽▽▽▽▽▽▽   Daily totals

Units of alcohol this week [ ]   Total alcohol kJ/Cal [ ]

Vitamins and supplements

	Fat	Protein	Carbs	Fibre	kJ/Cal
WEEKLY TOTALS					

WEEKLY PERSONAL SUMMARY

Mood 1 2 3 4 5 ○○○○○   **Appetite** 1 2 3 4 5 ○○○○○

Energy level 1 2 3 4 5 ○○○○○   **Stress level** 1 2 3 4 5 ○○○○○

Hours of sleep [ ]   **Sleep quality** 1 2 3 4 5 ○○○○○

kJ/Cal intake

Planned kJ/Cal	
Actual kJ/Cal	

Difference [+/-]

Weight at end of week

BMI at end of week

Injuries or illnesses

116

EXERCISE DIARY

STRENGTH TRAINING		SET 1		SET 2		SET 3		SET4			
Exercise	Focus area	Reps	Weight	Reps	Weight	Reps	Weight	Reps	Weight	Equipment	Ease

CARDIO TRAINING

Exercise	Time	Distance	Intensity	Heart rate	Ease	kJ/Cal burnt

Total kJ/Cal burnt

INCIDENTAL EXERCISE

Day	Activity	Day	Activity

WEEK BEGINNING ___ / ___ / ___

Weight at start of week [____]

BMI at start of week [____]

Planned kJ/Cal this week [____]

Possible diet-busting occasions this week

[____]

Planned exercise sessions this week

	Exercise	Completed [Y/N]
Monday		
Tuesday		
Wednesday		
Thursday		
Friday		
Saturday		
Sunday		

FOOD DIARY

MONDAY

	Time		Quantity	Fat	Protein	Carbs	Fibre	kJ/Cal
Breakfast 1 2 3 4 5 ○○○○○ HUNGER SCALE								
Mid-morning ○○○○○								
Lunch 1 2 3 4 5 ○○○○○ HUNGER SCALE								
Mid-afternoon ○○○○○								
Dinner 1 2 3 4 5 ○○○○○ HUNGER SCALE								
Evening ○○○○○								

Coffees/teas [____] Fluid intake ▽▽▽▽▽▽▽▽▽▽ Daily totals

TUESDAY

	Time		Quantity	Fat	Protein	Carbs	Fibre	kJ/Cal
Breakfast 1 2 3 4 5 ○○○○○ HUNGER SCALE								
Mid-morning ○○○○○								
Lunch 1 2 3 4 5 ○○○○○ HUNGER SCALE								
Mid-afternoon ○○○○○								
Dinner 1 2 3 4 5 ○○○○○ HUNGER SCALE								
Evening ○○○○○								

Coffees/teas [____] Fluid intake ▽▽▽▽▽▽▽▽▽▽ Daily totals

WEDNESDAY

	Time			Quantity	Fat	Protein	Carbs	Fibre	kJ/Cal
Breakfast 1 2 3 4 5 ○○○○○ HUNGER SCALE									
Mid-morning ○○○○○									
Lunch 1 2 3 4 5 ○○○○○ HUNGER SCALE									
Mid-afternoon ○○○○○									
Dinner 1 2 3 4 5 ○○○○○ HUNGER SCALE									
Evening ○○○○○									

Coffees/teas ☐   Fluid intake ▽▽▽▽▽▽▽▽▽▽   Daily totals

THURSDAY

	Time			Quantity	Fat	Protein	Carbs	Fibre	kJ/Cal
Breakfast 1 2 3 4 5 ○○○○○ HUNGER SCALE									
Mid-morning ○○○○○									
Lunch 1 2 3 4 5 ○○○○○ HUNGER SCALE									
Mid-afternoon ○○○○○									
Dinner 1 2 3 4 5 ○○○○○ HUNGER SCALE									
Evening ○○○○○									

Coffees/teas   Fluid intake ▽▽▽▽▽▽▽▽▽▽   Daily totals

FRIDAY

	Time			Quantity	Fat	Protein	Carbs	Fibre	kJ/Cal
Breakfast 1 2 3 4 5 ○○○○○ HUNGER SCALE									
Mid-morning ○○○○○									
Lunch 1 2 3 4 5 ○○○○○ HUNGER SCALE									
Mid-afternoon ○○○○○									
Dinner 1 2 3 4 5 ○○○○○ HUNGER SCALE									
Evening ○○○○○									

Coffees/teas   Fluid intake ▽▽▽▽▽▽▽▽▽▽   Daily totals

SATURDAY

	Time							Quantity	Fat	Protein	Carbs	Fibre	kJ/Cal
Breakfast 1 2 3 4 5 ○ ○ ○ ○ ○ HUNGER SCALE													
Mid-morning ○ ○ ○ ○ ○													
Lunch 1 2 3 4 5 ○ ○ ○ ○ ○ HUNGER SCALE													
Mid-afternoon ○ ○ ○ ○ ○													
Dinner 1 2 3 4 5 ○ ○ ○ ○ ○ HUNGER SCALE													
Evening ○ ○ ○ ○ ○													

Coffees/teas ▢   Fluid intake ⊔ ⊔ ⊔ ⊔ ⊔ ⊔ ⊔ ⊔ ⊔ ⊔   Daily totals

SUNDAY

	Time							Quantity	Fat	Protein	Carbs	Fibre	kJ/Cal
Breakfast 1 2 3 4 5 ○ ○ ○ ○ ○ HUNGER SCALE													
Mid-morning ○ ○ ○ ○ ○													
Lunch 1 2 3 4 5 ○ ○ ○ ○ ○ HUNGER SCALE													
Mid-afternoon ○ ○ ○ ○ ○													
Dinner 1 2 3 4 5 ○ ○ ○ ○ ○ HUNGER SCALE													
Evening ○ ○ ○ ○ ○													

Coffees/teas ▢   Fluid intake ⊔ ⊔ ⊔ ⊔ ⊔ ⊔ ⊔ ⊔ ⊔ ⊔   Daily totals

Units of alcohol this week ▢   Total alcohol kJ/Cal

Vitamins and supplements

WEEKLY TOTALS	Fat	Protein	Carbs	Fibre	kJ/Cal

WEEKLY PERSONAL SUMMARY

Mood 1 2 3 4 5 ○ ○ ○ ○ ○   **Appetite** 1 2 3 4 5 ○ ○ ○ ○ ○

Energy level 1 2 3 4 5 ○ ○ ○ ○ ○   **Stress level** 1 2 3 4 5 ○ ○ ○ ○ ○

Hours of sleep ▢   **Sleep quality** 1 2 3 4 5 ○ ○ ○ ○ ○

kJ/Cal intake	
Planned kJ/Cal	
Actual kJ/Cal	
Difference [+/-]	

Weight at end of week ▢

BMI at end of week

Injuries or illnesses

EXERCISE DIARY

STRENGTH TRAINING

Exercise	Focus area	SET 1 Reps	SET 1 Weight	SET 2 Reps	SET 2 Weight	SET 3 Reps	SET 3 Weight	SET4 Reps	SET4 Weight	Equipment	Ease

CARDIO TRAINING

Exercise	Time	Distance	Intensity	Heart rate	Ease	kJ/Cal burnt

Total kJ/Cal burnt

INCIDENTAL EXERCISE

Day	Activity	Day	Activity

WEEK BEGINNING ___ / ___ / ___

Weight at start of week [ ]

BMI at start of week [ ]

Planned kJ/Cal this week [ ]

Possible diet-busting occasions this week

Planned exercise sessions this week

	Exercise	Completed [Y/N]
Monday		
Tuesday		
Wednesday		
Thursday		
Friday		
Saturday		
Sunday		

FOOD DIARY

MONDAY

	Time		Quantity	Fat	Protein	Carbs	Fibre	kJ/Cal
Breakfast 1 2 3 4 5 ○○○○○ HUNGER SCALE								
Mid-morning ○○○○○								
Lunch 1 2 3 4 5 ○○○○○ HUNGER SCALE								
Mid-afternoon ○○○○○								
Dinner 1 2 3 4 5 ○○○○○ HUNGER SCALE								
Evening ○○○○○								

Coffees/teas [ ] Fluid intake ▭▭▭▭▭▭▭▭▭▭ Daily totals

TUESDAY

	Time		Quantity	Fat	Protein	Carbs	Fibre	kJ/Cal
Breakfast 1 2 3 4 5 ○○○○○ HUNGER SCALE								
Mid-morning ○○○○○								
Lunch 1 2 3 4 5 ○○○○○ HUNGER SCALE								
Mid-afternoon ○○○○○								
Dinner 1 2 3 4 5 ○○○○○ HUNGER SCALE								
Evening ○○○○○								

Coffees/teas [ ] Fluid intake ▭▭▭▭▭▭▭▭▭▭ Daily totals

WEDNESDAY

	Time						Quantity	Fat	Protein	Carbs	Fibre	kJ/Cal

Breakfast
1 2 3 4 5
○ ○ ○ ○ ○
HUNGER SCALE

Mid-morning
○ ○ ○ ○ ○

Lunch
1 2 3 4 5
○ ○ ○ ○ ○
HUNGER SCALE

Mid-afternoon
○ ○ ○ ○ ○

Dinner
1 2 3 4 5
○ ○ ○ ○ ○
HUNGER SCALE

Evening
○ ○ ○ ○ ○

Coffees/teas ___ Fluid intake ▽▽▽▽▽▽▽▽▽▽ Daily totals

THURSDAY

Breakfast
1 2 3 4 5
○ ○ ○ ○ ○
HUNGER SCALE

Mid-morning
○ ○ ○ ○ ○

Lunch
1 2 3 4 5
○ ○ ○ ○ ○
HUNGER SCALE

Mid-afternoon
○ ○ ○ ○ ○

Dinner
1 2 3 4 5
○ ○ ○ ○ ○
HUNGER SCALE

Evening
○ ○ ○ ○ ○

Coffees/teas ___ Fluid intake ▽▽▽▽▽▽▽▽▽▽ Daily totals

FRIDAY

Breakfast
1 2 3 4 5
○ ○ ○ ○ ○
HUNGER SCALE

Mid-morning
○ ○ ○ ○ ○

Lunch
1 2 3 4 5
○ ○ ○ ○ ○
HUNGER SCALE

Mid-afternoon
○ ○ ○ ○ ○

Dinner
1 2 3 4 5
○ ○ ○ ○ ○
HUNGER SCALE

Evening
○ ○ ○ ○ ○

Coffees/teas ___ Fluid intake ▽▽▽▽▽▽▽▽▽▽ Daily totals

123

SATURDAY

	Time		Quantity	Fat	Protein	Carbs	Fibre	kJ/Cal
Breakfast 1 2 3 4 5 ○○○○○ HUNGER SCALE								
Mid-morning ○○○○○								
Lunch 1 2 3 4 5 ○○○○○ HUNGER SCALE								
Mid-afternoon ○○○○○								
Dinner 1 2 3 4 5 ○○○○○ HUNGER SCALE								
Evening ○○○○○								

Coffees/teas ☐   Fluid intake ▽▽▽▽▽▽▽▽▽▽   Daily totals

SUNDAY

	Time		Quantity	Fat	Protein	Carbs	Fibre	kJ/Cal
Breakfast 1 2 3 4 5 ○○○○○ HUNGER SCALE								
Mid-morning ○○○○○								
Lunch 1 2 3 4 5 ○○○○○ HUNGER SCALE								
Mid-afternoon ○○○○○								
Dinner 1 2 3 4 5 ○○○○○ HUNGER SCALE								
Evening ○○○○○								

Coffees/teas ☐   Fluid intake ▽▽▽▽▽▽▽▽▽▽   Daily totals

Units of alcohol this week ☐   Total alcohol kJ/Cal ☐

Vitamins and supplements

WEEKLY TOTALS	Fat	Protein	Carbs	Fibre	kJ/Cal

WEEKLY PERSONAL SUMMARY

Mood 1 2 3 4 5 ○○○○○   **Appetite** 1 2 3 4 5 ○○○○○

Energy level 1 2 3 4 5 ○○○○○   **Stress level** 1 2 3 4 5 ○○○○○

Hours of sleep ☐   **Sleep quality** 1 2 3 4 5 ○○○○○

kJ/Cal intake

Planned kJ/Cal	
Actual kJ/Cal	
Difference [+/-]	

Weight at end of week ☐

BMI at end of week ☐

Injuries or illnesses

EXERCISE DIARY

STRENGTH TRAINING		SET 1		SET 2		SET 3		SET 4			
Exercise	Focus area	Reps	Weight	Reps	Weight	Reps	Weight	Reps	Weight	Equipment	Ease

CARDIO TRAINING

Exercise	Time	Distance	Intensity	Heart rate	Ease	kJ/Cal burnt

Total kJ/Cal burnt

INCIDENTAL EXERCISE

Day	Activity	Day	Activity

WEEK BEGINNING ___ / ___ / ___

Weight at start of week ▢

BMI at start of week ▢

Planned kJ/Cal this week ▢

Possible diet-busting occasions this week

Planned exercise sessions this week

	Exercise	Completed [Y/N]
Monday		
Tuesday		
Wednesday		
Thursday		
Friday		
Saturday		
Sunday		

FOOD DIARY

MONDAY

	Time		Quantity	Fat	Protein	Carbs	Fibre	kJ/Cal
Breakfast 1 2 3 4 5 ○ ○ ○ ○ ○ HUNGER SCALE								
Mid-morning ○ ○ ○ ○ ○								
Lunch 1 2 3 4 5 ○ ○ ○ ○ ○ HUNGER SCALE								
Mid-afternoon ○ ○ ○ ○ ○								
Dinner 1 2 3 4 5 ○ ○ ○ ○ ○ HUNGER SCALE								
Evening ○ ○ ○ ○ ○								

Coffees/teas ▢   Fluid intake ▢▢▢▢▢▢▢▢▢▢   Daily totals

TUESDAY

	Time		Quantity	Fat	Protein	Carbs	Fibre	kJ/Cal
Breakfast 1 2 3 4 5 ○ ○ ○ ○ ○ HUNGER SCALE								
Mid-morning ○ ○ ○ ○ ○								
Lunch 1 2 3 4 5 ○ ○ ○ ○ ○ HUNGER SCALE								
Mid-afternoon ○ ○ ○ ○ ○								
Dinner 1 2 3 4 5 ○ ○ ○ ○ ○ HUNGER SCALE								
Evening ○ ○ ○ ○ ○								

Coffees/teas ▢   Fluid intake ▢▢▢▢▢▢▢▢▢▢   Daily totals

WEDNESDAY

	Time		Quantity	Fat	Protein	Carbs	Fibre	kJ/Cal
Breakfast 1 2 3 4 5 ○ ○ ○ ○ ○ HUNGER SCALE								
Mid-morning ○ ○ ○ ○ ○								
Lunch 1 2 3 4 5 ○ ○ ○ ○ ○ HUNGER SCALE								
Mid-afternoon ○ ○ ○ ○ ○								
Dinner 1 2 3 4 5 ○ ○ ○ ○ ○ HUNGER SCALE								
Evening ○ ○ ○ ○ ○								

Coffees/teas   Fluid intake ▽▽▽▽▽▽▽▽▽▽   Daily totals

THURSDAY

	Time		Quantity	Fat	Protein	Carbs	Fibre	kJ/Cal
Breakfast 1 2 3 4 5 ○ ○ ○ ○ ○ HUNGER SCALE								
Mid-morning ○ ○ ○ ○ ○								
Lunch 1 2 3 4 5 ○ ○ ○ ○ ○ HUNGER SCALE								
Mid-afternoon ○ ○ ○ ○ ○								
Dinner 1 2 3 4 5 ○ ○ ○ ○ ○ HUNGER SCALE								
Evening ○ ○ ○ ○ ○								

Coffees/teas   Fluid intake ▽▽▽▽▽▽▽▽▽▽   Daily totals

FRIDAY

	Time		Quantity	Fat	Protein	Carbs	Fibre	kJ/Cal
Breakfast 1 2 3 4 5 ○ ○ ○ ○ ○ HUNGER SCALE								
Mid-morning ○ ○ ○ ○ ○								
Lunch 1 2 3 4 5 ○ ○ ○ ○ ○ HUNGER SCALE								
Mid-afternoon ○ ○ ○ ○ ○								
Dinner 1 2 3 4 5 ○ ○ ○ ○ ○ HUNGER SCALE								
Evening ○ ○ ○ ○ ○								

Coffees/teas   Fluid intake ▽▽▽▽▽▽▽▽▽▽   Daily totals

SATURDAY

	Time		Quantity	Fat	Protein	Carbs	Fibre	kJ/Cal
Breakfast 1 2 3 4 5 ○○○○○ HUNGER SCALE								
Mid-morning ○○○○○								
Lunch 1 2 3 4 5 ○○○○○ HUNGER SCALE								
Mid-afternoon ○○○○○								
Dinner 1 2 3 4 5 ○○○○○ HUNGER SCALE								
Evening ○○○○○								

Coffees/teas [ ]   Fluid intake ▽▽▽▽▽▽▽▽▽▽   Daily totals

SUNDAY

	Time		Quantity	Fat	Protein	Carbs	Fibre	kJ/Cal
Breakfast 1 2 3 4 5 ○○○○○ HUNGER SCALE								
Mid-morning ○○○○○								
Lunch 1 2 3 4 5 ○○○○○ HUNGER SCALE								
Mid-afternoon ○○○○○								
Dinner 1 2 3 4 5 ○○○○○ HUNGER SCALE								
Evening ○○○○○								

Coffees/teas [ ]   Fluid intake ▽▽▽▽▽▽▽▽▽▽   Daily totals

Units of alcohol this week [ ]   Total alcohol kJ/Cal [ ]

Vitamins and supplements

	Fat	Protein	Carbs	Fibre	kJ/Cal
WEEKLY TOTALS					

WEEKLY PERSONAL SUMMARY

Mood 1 2 3 4 5 ○○○○○   **Appetite** 1 2 3 4 5 ○○○○○

Energy level 1 2 3 4 5 ○○○○○   **Stress level** 1 2 3 4 5 ○○○○○

Hours of sleep [ ]   **Sleep quality** 1 2 3 4 5 ○○○○○

kJ/Cal intake

Planned kJ/Cal	
Actual kJ/Cal	

Difference [+/-] [ ]

Weight at end of week [ ]

BMI at end of week [ ]

Injuries or illnesses

128

EXERCISE DIARY

STRENGTH TRAINING		SET 1		SET 2		SET 3		SET4			
Exercise	Focus area	Reps	Weight	Reps	Weight	Reps	Weight	Reps	Weight	Equipment	Ease

CARDIO TRAINING

Exercise	Time	Distance	Intensity	Heart rate	Ease	kJ/Cal burnt

Total kJ/Cal burnt

INCIDENTAL EXERCISE

Day	Activity	Day	Activity

WEEK BEGINNING ___ / ___ / ___

Weight at start of week [ ]

BMI at start of week [ ]

Planned kJ/Cal this week [ ]

Possible diet-busting occasions this week

[ ]

Planned exercise sessions this week

	Exercise	Completed [Y/N]
Monday		
Tuesday		
Wednesday		
Thursday		
Friday		
Saturday		
Sunday		

FOOD DIARY

MONDAY

	Time		Quantity	Fat	Protein	Carbs	Fibre	kJ/Cal
Breakfast 1 2 3 4 5 ○○○○○ HUNGER SCALE								
Mid-morning ○○○○○								
Lunch 1 2 3 4 5 ○○○○○ HUNGER SCALE								
Mid-afternoon ○○○○○								
Dinner 1 2 3 4 5 ○○○○○ HUNGER SCALE								
Evening ○○○○								

Coffees/teas [ ] Fluid intake ▽▽▽▽▽▽▽▽▽▽ Daily totals

TUESDAY

	Time		Quantity	Fat	Protein	Carbs	Fibre	kJ/Cal
Breakfast 1 2 3 4 5 ○○○○○ HUNGER SCALE								
Mid-morning ○○○○○								
Lunch 1 2 3 4 5 ○○○○○ HUNGER SCALE								
Mid-afternoon ○○○○○								
Dinner 1 2 3 4 5 ○○○○○ HUNGER SCALE								
Evening ○○○○○								

Coffees/teas [ ] Fluid intake ▽▽▽▽▽▽▽▽▽▽ Daily totals

WEDNESDAY

	Time		Quantity	Fat	Protein	Carbs	Fibre	kJ/Cal
Breakfast 1 2 3 4 5 ○ ○ ○ ○ ○ HUNGER SCALE								
Mid-morning ○ ○ ○ ○ ○								
Lunch 1 2 3 4 5 ○ ○ ○ ○ ○ HUNGER SCALE								
Mid-afternoon ○ ○ ○ ○ ○								
Dinner 1 2 3 4 5 ○ ○ ○ ○ ○ HUNGER SCALE								
Evening ○ ○ ○ ○ ○								

Coffees/teas   Fluid intake ∪ ∪ ∪ ∪ ∪ ∪ ∪ ∪ ∪ ∪   Daily totals

THURSDAY

	Time		Quantity	Fat	Protein	Carbs	Fibre	kJ/Cal
Breakfast 1 2 3 4 5 ○ ○ ○ ○ ○ HUNGER SCALE								
Mid-morning ○ ○ ○ ○ ○								
Lunch 1 2 3 4 5 ○ ○ ○ ○ ○ HUNGER SCALE								
Mid-afternoon ○ ○ ○ ○ ○								
Dinner 1 2 3 4 5 ○ ○ ○ ○ ○ HUNGER SCALE								
Evening ○ ○ ○ ○ ○								

Coffees/teas   Fluid intake ∪ ∪ ∪ ∪ ∪ ∪ ∪ ∪ ∪ ∪   Daily totals

FRIDAY

	Time		Quantity	Fat	Protein	Carbs	Fibre	kJ/Cal
Breakfast 1 2 3 4 5 ○ ○ ○ ○ ○ HUNGER SCALE								
Mid-morning ○ ○ ○ ○ ○								
Lunch 1 2 3 4 5 ○ ○ ○ ○ ○ HUNGER SCALE								
Mid-afternoon ○ ○ ○ ○ ○								
Dinner 1 2 3 4 5 ○ ○ ○ ○ ○ HUNGER SCALE								
Evening ○ ○ ○ ○ ○								

Coffees/teas   Fluid intake ∪ ∪ ∪ ∪ ∪ ∪ ∪ ∪ ∪ ∪   Daily totals

SATURDAY

	Time		Quantity	Fat	Protein	Carbs	Fibre	kJ/Cal
Breakfast 1 2 3 4 5 ○ ○ ○ ○ ○ HUNGER SCALE								
Mid-morning ○ ○ ○ ○ ○								
Lunch 1 2 3 4 5 ○ ○ ○ ○ ○ HUNGER SCALE								
Mid-afternoon ○ ○ ○ ○ ○								
Dinner 1 2 3 4 5 ○ ○ ○ ○ ○ HUNGER SCALE								
Evening ○ ○ ○ ○ ○								

Coffees/teas [ ]   Fluid intake ▯▯▯▯▯▯▯▯▯▯   Daily totals

SUNDAY

	Time		Quantity	Fat	Protein	Carbs	Fibre	kJ/Cal
Breakfast 1 2 3 4 5 ○ ○ ○ ○ ○ HUNGER SCALE								
Mid-morning ○ ○ ○ ○ ○								
Lunch 1 2 3 4 5 ○ ○ ○ ○ ○ HUNGER SCALE								
Mid-afternoon ○ ○ ○ ○ ○								
Dinner 1 2 3 4 5 ○ ○ ○ ○ ○ HUNGER SCALE								
Evening ○ ○ ○ ○ ○								

Coffees/teas [ ]   Fluid intake ▯▯▯▯▯▯▯▯▯▯   Daily totals

Units of alcohol this week [ ]   Total alcohol kJ/Cal [ ]

Vitamins and supplements

WEEKLY TOTALS	Fat	Protein	Carbs	Fibre	kJ/Cal

WEEKLY PERSONAL SUMMARY

Mood 1 2 3 4 5 ○ ○ ○ ○ ○   **Appetite** 1 2 3 4 5 ○ ○ ○ ○ ○

Energy level 1 2 3 4 5 ○ ○ ○ ○ ○   **Stress level** 1 2 3 4 5 ○ ○ ○ ○ ○

Hours of sleep [ ]   **Sleep quality** 1 2 3 4 5 ○ ○ ○ ○ ○

kJ/Cal intake

Planned kJ/Cal	
Actual kJ/Cal	

Difference [+/-]

Weight at end of week

BMI at end of week

Injuries or illnesses

EXERCISE DIARY

STRENGTH TRAINING		SET 1		SET 2		SET 3		SET4			
Exercise	Focus area	Reps	Weight	Reps	Weight	Reps	Weight	Reps	Weight	Equipment	Ease

CARDIO TRAINING

Exercise	Time	Distance	Intensity	Heart rate	Ease	kJ/Cal burnt

Total kJ/Cal burnt

INCIDENTAL EXERCISE

Day	Activity	Day	Activity

WEEK BEGINNING ___ / ___ / ___

Weight at start of week ___

BMI at start of week ___

Planned kJ/Cal this week ___

Possible diet-busting occasions this week

Planned exercise sessions this week

	Exercise	Completed [Y/N]
Monday		
Tuesday		
Wednesday		
Thursday		
Friday		
Saturday		
Sunday		

FOOD DIARY

MONDAY

	Time		Quantity	Fat	Protein	Carbs	Fibre	kJ/Cal
Breakfast 1 2 3 4 5 ○○○○○ HUNGER SCALE								
Mid-morning ○○○○○								
Lunch 1 2 3 4 5 ○○○○○ HUNGER SCALE								
Mid-afternoon ○○○○○								
Dinner 1 2 3 4 5 ○○○○○ HUNGER SCALE								
Evening ○○○○○								

Coffees/teas ___ Fluid intake ☐☐☐☐☐☐☐☐☐☐ Daily totals

TUESDAY

	Time		Quantity	Fat	Protein	Carbs	Fibre	kJ/Cal
Breakfast 1 2 3 4 5 ○○○○○ HUNGER SCALE								
Mid-morning ○○○○○								
Lunch 1 2 3 4 5 ○○○○○ HUNGER SCALE								
Mid-afternoon ○○○○○								
Dinner 1 2 3 4 5 ○○○○○ HUNGER SCALE								
Evening ○○○○○								

Coffees/teas ___ Fluid intake ☐☐☐☐☐☐☐☐☐☐ Daily totals

WEDNESDAY

	Time		Quantity	Fat	Protein	Carbs	Fibre	kJ/Cal
Breakfast 1 2 3 4 5 ○ ○ ○ ○ ○ HUNGER SCALE								
Mid-morning ○ ○ ○ ○ ○								
Lunch 1 2 3 4 5 ○ ○ ○ ○ ○ HUNGER SCALE								
Mid-afternoon ○ ○ ○ ○ ○								
Dinner 1 2 3 4 5 ○ ○ ○ ○ ○ HUNGER SCALE								
Evening ○ ○ ○ ○ ○								

Coffees/teas   Fluid intake ▽▽▽▽▽▽▽▽▽▽   Daily totals

THURSDAY

	Time		Quantity	Fat	Protein	Carbs	Fibre	kJ/Cal
Breakfast 1 2 3 4 5 ○ ○ ○ ○ ○ HUNGER SCALE								
Mid-morning ○ ○ ○ ○ ○								
Lunch 1 2 3 4 5 ○ ○ ○ ○ ○ HUNGER SCALE								
Mid-afternoon ○ ○ ○ ○ ○								
Dinner 1 2 3 4 5 ○ ○ ○ ○ ○ HUNGER SCALE								
Evening ○ ○ ○ ○ ○								

Coffees/teas   Fluid intake ▽▽▽▽▽▽▽▽▽▽   Daily totals

FRIDAY

	Time		Quantity	Fat	Protein	Carbs	Fibre	kJ/Cal
Breakfast 1 2 3 4 5 ○ ○ ○ ○ ○ HUNGER SCALE								
Mid-morning ○ ○ ○ ○ ○								
Lunch 1 2 3 4 5 ○ ○ ○ ○ ○ HUNGER SCALE								
Mid-afternoon ○ ○ ○ ○ ○								
Dinner 1 2 3 4 5 ○ ○ ○ ○ ○ HUNGER SCALE								
Evening ○ ○ ○ ○ ○								

Coffees/teas   Fluid intake ▽▽▽▽▽▽▽▽▽▽   Daily totals

SATURDAY

	Time				Quantity	Fat	Protein	Carbs	Fibre	kJ/Cal
Breakfast 1 2 3 4 5 ○ ○ ○ ○ ○ HUNGER SCALE										
Mid-morning ○ ○ ○ ○ ○										
Lunch 1 2 3 4 5 ○ ○ ○ ○ ○ HUNGER SCALE										
Mid-afternoon ○ ○ ○ ○ ○										
Dinner 1 2 3 4 5 ○ ○ ○ ○ ○ HUNGER SCALE										
Evening ○ ○ ○ ○ ○										

Coffees/teas [ ]   Fluid intake ⊔ ⊔ ⊔ ⊔ ⊔ ⊔ ⊔ ⊔ ⊔ ⊔   Daily totals

SUNDAY

	Time				Quantity	Fat	Protein	Carbs	Fibre	kJ/Cal
Breakfast 1 2 3 4 5 ○ ○ ○ ○ ○ HUNGER SCALE										
Mid-morning ○ ○ ○ ○ ○										
Lunch 1 2 3 4 5 ○ ○ ○ ○ ○ HUNGER SCALE										
Mid-afternoon ○ ○ ○ ○ ○										
Dinner 1 2 3 4 5 ○ ○ ○ ○ ○ HUNGER SCALE										
Evening ○ ○ ○ ○ ○										

Coffees/teas [ ]   Fluid intake ⊔ ⊔ ⊔ ⊔ ⊔ ⊔ ⊔ ⊔ ⊔ ⊔   Daily totals

Units of alcohol this week [ ]   Total alcohol kJ/Cal [ ]

Vitamins and supplements

WEEKLY TOTALS	Fat	Protein	Carbs	Fibre	kJ/Cal

WEEKLY PERSONAL SUMMARY

Mood 1 2 3 4 5 ○ ○ ○ ○ ○   **Appetite** 1 2 3 4 5 ○ ○ ○ ○ ○

Energy level 1 2 3 4 5 ○ ○ ○ ○ ○   **Stress level** 1 2 3 4 5 ○ ○ ○ ○ ○

Hours of sleep [ ]   **Sleep quality** 1 2 3 4 5 ○ ○ ○ ○ ○

Injuries or illnesses

kJ/Cal intake

Planned kJ/Cal	
Actual kJ/Cal	

Difference [+/-]

Weight at end of week

BMI at end of week

EXERCISE DIARY

STRENGTH TRAINING		SET 1		SET 2		SET 3		SET4			
Exercise	Focus area	Reps	Weight	Reps	Weight	Reps	Weight	Reps	Weight	Equipment	Ease

CARDIO TRAINING

Exercise	Time	Distance	Intensity	Heart rate	Ease	kJ/Cal burnt

Total kJ/Cal burnt

INCIDENTAL EXERCISE

Day	Activity	Day	Activity

WEEK BEGINNING   /   /

Weight at start of week

BMI at start of week

Planned kJ/Cal this week

Possible diet-busting occasions this week

Planned exercise sessions this week

	Exercise	Completed [Y/N]
Monday		
Tuesday		
Wednesday		
Thursday		
Friday		
Saturday		
Sunday		

FOOD DIARY

MONDAY

Time		Quantity	Fat	Protein	Carbs	Fibre	kJ/Cal
Breakfast 1 2 3 4 5 ○○○○○ HUNGER SCALE							
Mid-morning ○○○○○							
Lunch 1 2 3 4 5 ○○○○○ HUNGER SCALE							
Mid-afternoon ○○○○○							
Dinner 1 2 3 4 5 ○○○○○ HUNGER SCALE							
Evening ○○○○○							

Coffees/teas   Fluid intake ▽▽▽▽▽▽▽▽▽▽▽▽ Daily totals

TUESDAY

Time		Quantity	Fat	Protein	Carbs	Fibre	kJ/Cal
Breakfast 1 2 3 4 5 ○○○○○ HUNGER SCALE							
Mid-morning ○○○○○							
Lunch 1 2 3 4 5 ○○○○○ HUNGER SCALE							
Mid-afternoon ○○○○○							
Dinner 1 2 3 4 5 ○○○○○ HUNGER SCALE							
Evening ○○○○○							

Coffees/teas   Fluid intake ▽▽▽▽▽▽▽▽▽▽▽▽ Daily totals

WEDNESDAY

	Time				Quantity	Fat	Protein	Carbs	Fibre	kJ/Cal
Breakfast 1 2 3 4 5 ○ ○ ○ ○ ○ HUNGER SCALE										
Mid-morning ○ ○ ○ ○ ○										
Lunch 1 2 3 4 5 ○ ○ ○ ○ ○ HUNGER SCALE										
Mid-afternoon ○ ○ ○ ○ ○										
Dinner 1 2 3 4 5 ○ ○ ○ ○ ○ HUNGER SCALE										
Evening ○ ○ ○ ○ ○										

Coffees/teas ___ Fluid intake ▽▽▽▽▽▽▽▽▽▽ Daily totals

THURSDAY

					Quantity	Fat	Protein	Carbs	Fibre	kJ/Cal
Breakfast 1 2 3 4 5 ○ ○ ○ ○ ○ HUNGER SCALE										
Mid-morning ○ ○ ○ ○ ○										
Lunch 1 2 3 4 5 ○ ○ ○ ○ ○ HUNGER SCALE										
Mid-afternoon ○ ○ ○ ○ ○										
Dinner 1 2 3 4 5 ○ ○ ○ ○ ○ HUNGER SCALE										
Evening ○ ○ ○ ○ ○										

Coffees/teas ___ Fluid intake ▽▽▽▽▽▽▽▽▽▽ Daily totals

FRIDAY

					Quantity	Fat	Protein	Carbs	Fibre	kJ/Cal
Breakfast 1 2 3 4 5 ○ ○ ○ ○ ○ HUNGER SCALE										
Mid-morning ○ ○ ○ ○ ○										
Lunch 1 2 3 4 5 ○ ○ ○ ○ ○ HUNGER SCALE										
Mid-afternoon ○ ○ ○ ○ ○										
Dinner 1 2 3 4 5 ○ ○ ○ ○ ○ HUNGER SCALE										
Evening ○ ○ ○ ○ ○										

Coffees/teas ___ Fluid intake ▽▽▽▽▽▽▽▽▽▽ Daily totals

139

SATURDAY

	Time		Quantity	Fat	Protein	Carbs	Fibre	kJ/Cal
Breakfast 1 2 3 4 5 ○○○○○ HUNGER SCALE								
Mid-morning ○○○○○								
Lunch 1 2 3 4 5 ○○○○○ HUNGER SCALE								
Mid-afternoon ○○○○○								
Dinner 1 2 3 4 5 ○○○○○ HUNGER SCALE								
Evening ○○○○○								
Coffees/teas		Fluid intake ⛾⛾⛾⛾⛾⛾⛾⛾⛾⛾	Daily totals					

SUNDAY

	Time		Quantity	Fat	Protein	Carbs	Fibre	kJ/Cal
Breakfast 1 2 3 4 5 ○○○○○ HUNGER SCALE								
Mid-morning ○○○○○								
Lunch 1 2 3 4 5 ○○○○○ HUNGER SCALE								
Mid-afternoon ○○○○○								
Dinner 1 2 3 4 5 ○○○○○ HUNGER SCALE								
Evening ○○○○○								
Coffees/teas		Fluid intake ⛾⛾⛾⛾⛾⛾⛾⛾⛾⛾	Daily totals					

Units of alcohol this week   **Total alcohol kJ/Cal**

Vitamins and supplements

	Fat	Protein	Carbs	Fibre	kJ/Cal
WEEKLY TOTALS					

WEEKLY PERSONAL SUMMARY

Mood 1 2 3 4 5 ○○○○○   **Appetite** 1 2 3 4 5 ○○○○○

Energy level 1 2 3 4 5 ○○○○○   **Stress level** 1 2 3 4 5 ○○○○○

Hours of sleep   **Sleep quality** 1 2 3 4 5 ○○○○○

Injuries or illnesses

kJ/Cal intake

Planned kJ/Cal	
Actual kJ/Cal	
Difference [+/-]	

Weight at end of week

BMI at end of week

EXERCISE DIARY

STRENGTH TRAINING		SET 1		SET 2		SET 3		SET4			
Exercise	Focus area	Reps	Weight	Reps	Weight	Reps	Weight	Reps	Weight	Equipment	Ease

CARDIO TRAINING

Exercise	Time	Distance	Intensity	Heart rate	Ease	kJ/Cal burnt

Total kJ/Cal burnt

INCIDENTAL EXERCISE

Day	Activity	Day	Activity

WEEK BEGINNING ___ / ___ / ___

Weight at start of week ▢

BMI at start of week ▢

Planned kJ/Cal this week ▢

Possible diet-busting occasions this week

▢

Planned exercise sessions this week

	Exercise	Completed [Y/N]
Monday		
Tuesday		
Wednesday		
Thursday		
Friday		
Saturday		
Sunday		

FOOD DIARY

MONDAY

	Time			Quantity	Fat	Protein	Carbs	Fibre	kJ/Cal
Breakfast 1 2 3 4 5 ○ ○ ○ ○ ○ HUNGER SCALE									
Mid-morning ○ ○ ○ ○ ○									
Lunch 1 2 3 4 5 ○ ○ ○ ○ ○ HUNGER SCALE									
Mid-afternoon ○ ○ ○ ○ ○									
Dinner 1 2 3 4 5 ○ ○ ○ ○ ○ HUNGER SCALE									
Evening ○ ○ ○ ○ ○									

Coffees/teas ▢   Fluid intake ▢▢▢▢▢▢▢▢▢▢   Daily totals

TUESDAY

	Time			Quantity	Fat	Protein	Carbs	Fibre	kJ/Cal
Breakfast 1 2 3 4 5 ○ ○ ○ ○ ○ HUNGER SCALE									
Mid-morning ○ ○ ○ ○ ○									
Lunch 1 2 3 4 5 ○ ○ ○ ○ ○ HUNGER SCALE									
Mid-afternoon ○ ○ ○ ○ ○									
Dinner 1 2 3 4 5 ○ ○ ○ ○ ○ HUNGER SCALE									
Evening ○ ○ ○ ○ ○									

Coffees/teas ▢   Fluid intake ▢▢▢▢▢▢▢▢▢▢   Daily totals

WEDNESDAY

	Time		Quantity	Fat	Protein	Carbs	Fibre	kJ/Cal
Breakfast 1 2 3 4 5 ○ ○ ○ ○ ○ HUNGER SCALE								
Mid-morning ○ ○ ○ ○ ○								
Lunch 1 2 3 4 5 ○ ○ ○ ○ ○ HUNGER SCALE								
Mid-afternoon ○ ○ ○ ○ ○								
Dinner 1 2 3 4 5 ○ ○ ○ ○ ○ HUNGER SCALE								
Evening ○ ○ ○ ○ ○								

Coffees/teas   Fluid intake ☐ ☐ ☐ ☐ ☐ ☐ ☐ ☐ ☐ ☐   Daily totals

THURSDAY

Breakfast 1 2 3 4 5 ○ ○ ○ ○ ○ HUNGER SCALE								
Mid-morning ○ ○ ○ ○ ○								
Lunch 1 2 3 4 5 ○ ○ ○ ○ ○ HUNGER SCALE								
Mid-afternoon ○ ○ ○ ○ ○								
Dinner 1 2 3 4 5 ○ ○ ○ ○ ○ HUNGER SCALE								
Evening ○ ○ ○ ○ ○								

Coffees/teas   Fluid intake ☐ ☐ ☐ ☐ ☐ ☐ ☐ ☐ ☐ ☐   Daily totals

FRIDAY

Breakfast 1 2 3 4 5 ○ ○ ○ ○ ○ HUNGER SCALE								
Mid-morning ○ ○ ○ ○ ○								
Lunch 1 2 3 4 5 ○ ○ ○ ○ ○ HUNGER SCALE								
Mid-afternoon ○ ○ ○ ○ ○								
Dinner 1 2 3 4 5 ○ ○ ○ ○ ○ HUNGER SCALE								
Evening ○ ○ ○ ○ ○								

Coffees/teas   Fluid intake ☐ ☐ ☐ ☐ ☐ ☐ ☐ ☐ ☐ ☐   Daily totals

SATURDAY

	Time		Quantity	Fat	Protein	Carbs	Fibre	kJ/Cal
Breakfast 1 2 3 4 5 ○○○○○ HUNGER SCALE								
Mid-morning ○○○○○								
Lunch 1 2 3 4 5 ○○○○○ HUNGER SCALE								
Mid-afternoon ○○○○○								
Dinner 1 2 3 4 5 ○○○○○ HUNGER SCALE								
Evening ○○○○○								

Coffees/teas ▢   Fluid intake ▭▭▭▭▭▭▭▭▭   Daily totals

SUNDAY

	Time		Quantity	Fat	Protein	Carbs	Fibre	kJ/Cal
Breakfast 1 2 3 4 5 ○○○○○ HUNGER SCALE								
Mid-morning ○○○○○								
Lunch 1 2 3 4 5 ○○○○○ HUNGER SCALE								
Mid-afternoon ○○○○○								
Dinner 1 2 3 4 5 ○○○○○ HUNGER SCALE								
Evening ○○○○○								

Coffees/teas ▢   Fluid intake ▭▭▭▭▭▭▭▭▭   Daily totals

Units of alcohol this week ▢   Total alcohol kJ/Cal ▢

Vitamins and supplements

WEEKLY TOTALS	Fat	Protein	Carbs	Fibre	kJ/Cal

WEEKLY PERSONAL SUMMARY

Mood 1 2 3 4 5 ○○○○○   **Appetite** 1 2 3 4 5 ○○○○○

Energy level 1 2 3 4 5 ○○○○○   **Stress level** 1 2 3 4 5 ○○○○○

Hours of sleep ▢   **Sleep quality** 1 2 3 4 5 ○○○○○

kJ/Cal intake

Planned kJ/Cal	
Actual kJ/Cal	
Difference [+/-]	

Weight at end of week

BMI at end of week

Injuries or illnesses

EXERCISE DIARY

STRENGTH TRAINING

		SET 1		SET 2		SET 3		SET4			
Exercise	Focus area	Reps	Weight	Reps	Weight	Reps	Weight	Reps	Weight	Equipment	Ease

CARDIO TRAINING

Exercise	Time	Distance	Intensity	Heart rate	Ease	kJ/Cal burnt

Total kJ/Cal burnt

INCIDENTAL EXERCISE

Day	Activity	Day	Activity

WEEK BEGINNING ___ / ___ / ___

Weight at start of week ___

BMI at start of week ___

Planned kJ/Cal this week ___

Possible diet-busting occasions this week

Planned exercise sessions this week

	Exercise	Completed [Y/N]
Monday		
Tuesday		
Wednesday		
Thursday		
Friday		
Saturday		
Sunday		

FOOD DIARY

MONDAY

	Time		Quantity	Fat	Protein	Carbs	Fibre	kJ/Cal
Breakfast 1 2 3 4 5 ○○○○○ HUNGER SCALE								
Mid-morning ○○○○○								
Lunch 1 2 3 4 5 ○○○○○ HUNGER SCALE								
Mid-afternoon ○○○○○								
Dinner 1 2 3 4 5 ○○○○○ HUNGER SCALE								
Evening ○○○○○								

Coffees/teas ___   Fluid intake ▽▽▽▽▽▽▽▽▽▽   Daily totals

TUESDAY

	Time		Quantity	Fat	Protein	Carbs	Fibre	kJ/Cal
Breakfast 1 2 3 4 5 ○○○○○ HUNGER SCALE								
Mid-morning ○○○○○								
Lunch 1 2 3 4 5 ○○○○○ HUNGER SCALE								
Mid-afternoon ○○○○○								
Dinner 1 2 3 4 5 ○○○○○ HUNGER SCALE								
Evening ○○○○○								

Coffees/teas ___   Fluid intake ▽▽▽▽▽▽▽▽▽▽   Daily totals

WEDNESDAY

	Time		Quantity	Fat	Protein	Carbs	Fibre	kJ/Cal
Breakfast 1 2 3 4 5 ○○○○○ HUNGER SCALE								
Mid-morning ○○○○○								
Lunch 1 2 3 4 5 ○○○○○ HUNGER SCALE								
Mid-afternoon ○○○○○								
Dinner 1 2 3 4 5 ○○○○○ HUNGER SCALE								
Evening ○○○○○								

Coffees/teas _____ Fluid intake ⊔⊔⊔⊔⊔⊔⊔⊔⊔⊔ Daily totals

THURSDAY

Breakfast 1 2 3 4 5 ○○○○○ HUNGER SCALE								
Mid-morning ○○○○○								
Lunch 1 2 3 4 5 ○○○○○ HUNGER SCALE								
Mid-afternoon ○○○○○								
Dinner 1 2 3 4 5 ○○○○○ HUNGER SCALE								
Evening ○○○○○								

Coffees/teas _____ Fluid intake ⊔⊔⊔⊔⊔⊔⊔⊔⊔⊔ Daily totals

FRIDAY

Breakfast 1 2 3 4 5 ○○○○○ HUNGER SCALE								
Mid-morning ○○○○○								
Lunch 1 2 3 4 5 ○○○○○ HUNGER SCALE								
Mid-afternoon ○○○○○								
Dinner 1 2 3 4 5 ○○○○○ HUNGER SCALE								
Evening ○○○○○								

Coffees/teas _____ Fluid intake ⊔⊔⊔⊔⊔⊔⊔⊔⊔⊔ Daily totals

SATURDAY

	Time		Quantity	Fat	Protein	Carbs	Fibre	kJ/Cal
Breakfast 1 2 3 4 5 ○○○○○ HUNGER SCALE								
Mid-morning ○○○○○								
Lunch 1 2 3 4 5 ○○○○○ HUNGER SCALE								
Mid-afternoon ○○○○○								
Dinner 1 2 3 4 5 ○○○○○ HUNGER SCALE								
Evening ○○○○○								

Coffees/teas [ ] Fluid intake ⛾⛾⛾⛾⛾⛾⛾⛾⛾⛾ Daily totals

SUNDAY

	Time		Quantity	Fat	Protein	Carbs	Fibre	kJ/Cal
Breakfast 1 2 3 4 5 ○○○○○ HUNGER SCALE								
Mid-morning ○○○○○								
Lunch 1 2 3 4 5 ○○○○○ HUNGER SCALE								
Mid-afternoon ○○○○○								
Dinner 1 2 3 4 5 ○○○○○ HUNGER SCALE								
Evening ○○○○○								

Coffees/teas [ ] Fluid intake ⛾⛾⛾⛾⛾⛾⛾⛾⛾⛾ Daily totals

Units of alcohol this week [ ]   Total alcohol kJ/Cal [ ]

Vitamins and supplements

WEEKLY TOTALS	Fat	Protein	Carbs	Fibre	kJ/Cal

WEEKLY PERSONAL SUMMARY

Mood 1 2 3 4 5 ○○○○○   **Appetite** 1 2 3 4 5 ○○○○○

Energy level 1 2 3 4 5 ○○○○○   **Stress level** 1 2 3 4 5 ○○○○○

Hours of sleep [ ]   **Sleep quality** 1 2 3 4 5 ○○○○○

Injuries or illnesses

kJ/Cal intake

Planned kJ/Cal	
Actual kJ/Cal	

Difference [+/-]

Weight at end of week [ ]

BMI at end of week [ ]

EXERCISE DIARY

STRENGTH TRAINING

Exercise	Focus area	SET 1 Reps	SET 1 Weight	SET 2 Reps	SET 2 Weight	SET 3 Reps	SET 3 Weight	SET4 Reps	SET4 Weight	Equipment	Ease

CARDIO TRAINING

Exercise	Time	Distance	Intensity	Heart rate	Ease	kJ/Cal burnt

Total kJ/Cal burnt

INCIDENTAL EXERCISE

Day	Activity	Day	Activity

WEEK BEGINNING ___ / ___ / ___

Weight at start of week ___

BMI at start of week ___

Planned kJ/Cal this week ___

Possible diet-busting occasions this week

___

Planned exercise sessions this week

	Exercise	Completed [Y/N]
Monday		
Tuesday		
Wednesday		
Thursday		
Friday		
Saturday		
Sunday		

FOOD DIARY

MONDAY

	Time		Quantity	Fat	Protein	Carbs	Fibre	kJ/Cal
Breakfast 1 2 3 4 5 ○○○○○ HUNGER SCALE								
Mid-morning ○○○○○								
Lunch 1 2 3 4 5 ○○○○○ HUNGER SCALE								
Mid-afternoon ○○○○○								
Dinner 1 2 3 4 5 ○○○○○ HUNGER SCALE								
Evening ○○○○○								

Coffees/teas ___   Fluid intake ▽▽▽▽▽▽▽▽▽▽   Daily totals

TUESDAY

	Time		Quantity	Fat	Protein	Carbs	Fibre	kJ/Cal
Breakfast 1 2 3 4 5 ○○○○○ HUNGER SCALE								
Mid-morning ○○○○○								
Lunch 1 2 3 4 5 ○○○○○ HUNGER SCALE								
Mid-afternoon ○○○○○								
Dinner 1 2 3 4 5 ○○○○○ HUNGER SCALE								
Evening ○○○○○								

Coffees/teas ___   Fluid intake ▽▽▽▽▽▽▽▽▽▽   Daily totals

WEDNESDAY

	Time		Quantity	Fat	Protein	Carbs	Fibre	kJ/Cal
Breakfast								
1 2 3 4 5 ○○○○○ HUNGER SCALE								
Mid-morning ○○○○○								
Lunch								
1 2 3 4 5 ○○○○○ HUNGER SCALE								
Mid-afternoon ○○○○○								
Dinner								
1 2 3 4 5 ○○○○○ HUNGER SCALE								
Evening ○○○○○								

Coffees/teas [ ]   Fluid intake ☐☐☐☐☐☐☐☐☐☐   Daily totals

THURSDAY

	Time		Quantity	Fat	Protein	Carbs	Fibre	kJ/Cal
Breakfast								
1 2 3 4 5 ○○○○○ HUNGER SCALE								
Mid-morning ○○○○○								
Lunch								
1 2 3 4 5 ○○○○○ HUNGER SCALE								
Mid-afternoon ○○○○○								
Dinner								
1 2 3 4 5 ○○○○○ HUNGER SCALE								
Evening ○○○○○								

Coffees/teas [ ]   Fluid intake ☐☐☐☐☐☐☐☐☐☐   Daily totals

FRIDAY

	Time		Quantity	Fat	Protein	Carbs	Fibre	kJ/Cal
Breakfast								
1 2 3 4 5 ○○○○○ HUNGER SCALE								
Mid-morning ○○○○○								
Lunch								
1 2 3 4 5 ○○○○○ HUNGER SCALE								
Mid-afternoon ○○○○○								
Dinner								
1 2 3 4 5 ○○○○○ HUNGER SCALE								
Evening ○○○○○								

Coffees/teas [ ]   Fluid intake ☐☐☐☐☐☐☐☐☐☐   Daily totals

SATURDAY

	Time		Quantity	Fat	Protein	Carbs	Fibre	kJ/Cal
Breakfast 1 2 3 4 5 ○ ○ ○ ○ ○ HUNGER SCALE								
Mid-morning ○ ○ ○ ○ ○								
Lunch 1 2 3 4 5 ○ ○ ○ ○ ○ HUNGER SCALE								
Mid-afternoon ○ ○ ○ ○ ○								
Dinner 1 2 3 4 5 ○ ○ ○ ○ ○ HUNGER SCALE								
Evening ○ ○ ○ ○ ○								

Coffees/teas Fluid intake ▽▽▽▽▽▽▽▽▽▽ Daily totals

SUNDAY

	Time		Quantity	Fat	Protein	Carbs	Fibre	kJ/Cal
Breakfast 1 2 3 4 5 ○ ○ ○ ○ ○ HUNGER SCALE								
Mid-morning ○ ○ ○ ○ ○								
Lunch 1 2 3 4 5 ○ ○ ○ ○ ○ HUNGER SCALE								
Mid-afternoon ○ ○ ○ ○ ○								
Dinner 1 2 3 4 5 ○ ○ ○ ○ ○ HUNGER SCALE								
Evening ○ ○ ○ ○ ○								

Coffees/teas Fluid intake ▽▽▽▽▽▽▽▽▽▽ Daily totals

Units of alcohol this week   Total alcohol kJ/Cal

Vitamins and supplements

WEEKLY TOTALS	Fat	Protein	Carbs	Fibre	kJ/Cal

WEEKLY PERSONAL SUMMARY

Mood 1 2 3 4 5 ○ ○ ○ ○ ○   **Appetite** 1 2 3 4 5 ○ ○ ○ ○ ○

Energy level 1 2 3 4 5 ○ ○ ○ ○ ○   **Stress level** 1 2 3 4 5 ○ ○ ○ ○ ○

Hours of sleep   **Sleep quality** 1 2 3 4 5 ○ ○ ○ ○ ○

Injuries or illnesses

kJ/Cal intake	
Planned kJ/Cal	
Actual kJ/Cal	
Difference [+/-]	

Weight at end of week

BMI at end of week

EXERCISE DIARY

STRENGTH TRAINING		SET 1		SET 2		SET 3		SET4			
Exercise	Focus area	Reps	Weight	Reps	Weight	Reps	Weight	Reps	Weight	Equipment	Ease

CARDIO TRAINING

Exercise	Time	Distance	Intensity	Heart rate	Ease	kJ/Cal burnt

Total kJ/Cal burnt

INCIDENTAL EXERCISE

Day	Activity	Day	Activity

WEEK BEGINNING   /   /

Weight at start of week

BMI at start of week

Planned kJ/Cal this week

Possible diet-busting occasions this week

Planned exercise sessions this week

	Exercise	Completed [Y/N]
Monday		
Tuesday		
Wednesday		
Thursday		
Friday		
Saturday		
Sunday		

FOOD DIARY

MONDAY

	Time		Quantity	Fat	Protein	Carbs	Fibre	kJ/Cal
Breakfast 1 2 3 4 5 ○○○○○ HUNGER SCALE								
Mid-morning ○○○○○								
Lunch 1 2 3 4 5 ○○○○○ HUNGER SCALE								
Mid-afternoon ○○○○○								
Dinner 1 2 3 4 5 ○○○○○ HUNGER SCALE								
Evening ○○○○○								

Coffees/teas   Fluid intake ▽▽▽▽▽▽▽▽▽▽   Daily totals

TUESDAY

	Time		Quantity	Fat	Protein	Carbs	Fibre	kJ/Cal
Breakfast 1 2 3 4 5 ○○○○○ HUNGER SCALE								
Mid-morning ○○○○○								
Lunch 1 2 3 4 5 ○○○○○ HUNGER SCALE								
Mid-afternoon ○○○○○								
Dinner 1 2 3 4 5 ○○○○○ HUNGER SCALE								
Evening ○○○○○								

Coffees/teas   Fluid intake ▽▽▽▽▽▽▽▽▽▽   Daily totals

WEDNESDAY

	Time		Quantity	Fat	Protein	Carbs	Fibre	kJ/Cal
Breakfast 1 2 3 4 5 ○○○○○ HUNGER SCALE								
Mid-morning ○○○○○								
Lunch 1 2 3 4 5 ○○○○○ HUNGER SCALE								
Mid-afternoon ○○○○○								
Dinner 1 2 3 4 5 ○○○○○ HUNGER SCALE								
Evening ○○○○○								

Coffees/teas   Fluid intake ▽▽▽▽▽▽▽▽▽▽   Daily totals

THURSDAY

	Time		Quantity	Fat	Protein	Carbs	Fibre	kJ/Cal
Breakfast 1 2 3 4 5 ○○○○○ HUNGER SCALE								
Mid-morning ○○○○○								
Lunch 1 2 3 4 5 ○○○○○ HUNGER SCALE								
Mid-afternoon ○○○○○								
Dinner 1 2 3 4 5 ○○○○○ HUNGER SCALE								
Evening ○○○○○								

Coffees/teas   Fluid intake ▽▽▽▽▽▽▽▽▽▽   Daily totals

FRIDAY

	Time		Quantity	Fat	Protein	Carbs	Fibre	kJ/Cal
Breakfast 1 2 3 4 5 ○○○○○ HUNGER SCALE								
Mid-morning ○○○○○								
Lunch 1 2 3 4 5 ○○○○○ HUNGER SCALE								
Mid-afternoon ○○○○○								
Dinner 1 2 3 4 5 ○○○○○ HUNGER SCALE								
Evening ○○○○○								

Coffees/teas   Fluid intake ▽▽▽▽▽▽▽▽▽▽   Daily totals

SATURDAY

	Time		Quantity	Fat	Protein	Carbs	Fibre	kJ/Cal
Breakfast 1 2 3 4 5 ○○○○○ HUNGER SCALE								
Mid-morning ○○○○○								
Lunch 1 2 3 4 5 ○○○○○ HUNGER SCALE								
Mid-afternoon ○○○○○								
Dinner 1 2 3 4 5 ○○○○○ HUNGER SCALE								
Evening ○○○○○								

Coffees/teas ☐ Fluid intake ▽▽▽▽▽▽▽▽▽▽ Daily totals

SUNDAY

	Time		Quantity	Fat	Protein	Carbs	Fibre	kJ/Cal
Breakfast 1 2 3 4 5 ○○○○○ HUNGER SCALE								
Mid-morning ○○○○○								
Lunch 1 2 3 4 5 ○○○○○ HUNGER SCALE								
Mid-afternoon ○○○○○								
Dinner 1 2 3 4 5 ○○○○○ HUNGER SCALE								
Evening ○○○○○								

Coffees/teas ☐ Fluid intake ▽▽▽▽▽▽▽▽▽▽ Daily totals

Units of alcohol this week ☐   Total alcohol kJ/Cal ☐

Vitamins and supplements

WEEKLY TOTALS	Fat	Protein	Carbs	Fibre	kJ/Cal

WEEKLY PERSONAL SUMMARY

Mood 1 2 3 4 5 ○○○○○   **Appetite** 1 2 3 4 5 ○○○○○

Energy level 1 2 3 4 5 ○○○○○   **Stress level** 1 2 3 4 5 ○○○○○

Hours of sleep ☐   **Sleep quality** 1 2 3 4 5 ○○○○○

Injuries or illnesses

kJ/Cal intake

Planned kJ/Cal	
Actual kJ/Cal	
Difference [+/-]	

Weight at end of week

BMI at end of week

EXERCISE DIARY

STRENGTH TRAINING		SET 1		SET 2		SET 3		SET4			
Exercise	Focus area	Reps	Weight	Reps	Weight	Reps	Weight	Reps	Weight	Equipment	Ease

CARDIO TRAINING

Exercise	Time	Distance	Intensity	Heart rate	Ease	kJ/Cal burnt

Total kJ/Cal burnt

INCIDENTAL EXERCISE

Day	Activity	Day	Activity

WEEK BEGINNING   /   /

Weight at start of week

BMI at start of week

Planned kJ/Cal this week

Possible diet-busting occasions this week

Planned exercise sessions this week

	Exercise	Completed [Y/N]
Monday		
Tuesday		
Wednesday		
Thursday		
Friday		
Saturday		
Sunday		

FOOD DIARY

MONDAY

	Time			Quantity	Fat	Protein	Carbs	Fibre	kJ/Cal
Breakfast 1 2 3 4 5 ○ ○ ○ ○ ○ HUNGER SCALE									
Mid-morning ○ ○ ○ ○ ○									
Lunch 1 2 3 4 5 ○ ○ ○ ○ ○ HUNGER SCALE									
Mid-afternoon ○ ○ ○ ○ ○									
Dinner 1 2 3 4 5 ○ ○ ○ ○ ○ HUNGER SCALE									
Evening ○ ○ ○ ○ ○									

Coffees/teas   Fluid intake ⊔ ⊔ ⊔ ⊔ ⊔ ⊔ ⊔ ⊔ ⊔ ⊔   Daily totals

TUESDAY

				Quantity	Fat	Protein	Carbs	Fibre	kJ/Cal
Breakfast 1 2 3 4 5 ○ ○ ○ ○ ○ HUNGER SCALE									
Mid-morning ○ ○ ○ ○ ○									
Lunch 1 2 3 4 5 ○ ○ ○ ○ ○ HUNGER SCALE									
Mid-afternoon ○ ○ ○ ○ ○									
Dinner 1 2 3 4 5 ○ ○ ○ ○ ○ HUNGER SCALE									
Evening ○ ○ ○ ○ ○									

Coffees/teas   Fluid intake ⊔ ⊔ ⊔ ⊔ ⊔ ⊔ ⊔ ⊔ ⊔ ⊔   Daily totals

WEDNESDAY

	Time		Quantity	Fat	Protein	Carbs	Fibre	kJ/Cal
Breakfast 1 2 3 4 5 ○ ○ ○ ○ ○ HUNGER SCALE								
Mid-morning ○ ○ ○ ○ ○								
Lunch 1 2 3 4 5 ○ ○ ○ ○ ○ HUNGER SCALE								
Mid-afternoon ○ ○ ○ ○ ○								
Dinner 1 2 3 4 5 ○ ○ ○ ○ ○ HUNGER SCALE								
Evening ○ ○ ○ ○ ○								

Coffees/teas   Fluid intake ⊔⊔⊔⊔⊔⊔⊔⊔⊔⊔   Daily totals

THURSDAY

	Time		Quantity	Fat	Protein	Carbs	Fibre	kJ/Cal
Breakfast 1 2 3 4 5 ○ ○ ○ ○ ○ HUNGER SCALE								
Mid-morning ○ ○ ○ ○ ○								
Lunch 1 2 3 4 5 ○ ○ ○ ○ ○ HUNGER SCALE								
Mid-afternoon ○ ○ ○ ○ ○								
Dinner 1 2 3 4 5 ○ ○ ○ ○ ○ HUNGER SCALE								
Evening ○ ○ ○ ○ ○								

Coffees/teas   Fluid intake ⊔⊔⊔⊔⊔⊔⊔⊔⊔⊔   Daily totals

FRIDAY

	Time		Quantity	Fat	Protein	Carbs	Fibre	kJ/Cal
Breakfast 1 2 3 4 5 ○ ○ ○ ○ ○ HUNGER SCALE								
Mid-morning ○ ○ ○ ○ ○								
Lunch 1 2 3 4 5 ○ ○ ○ ○ ○ HUNGER SCALE								
Mid-afternoon ○ ○ ○ ○ ○								
Dinner 1 2 3 4 5 ○ ○ ○ ○ ○ HUNGER SCALE								
Evening ○ ○ ○ ○ ○								

Coffees/teas   Fluid intake ⊔⊔⊔⊔⊔⊔⊔⊔⊔⊔   Daily totals

SATURDAY

	Time		Quantity	Fat	Protein	Carbs	Fibre	kJ/Cal
Breakfast 1 2 3 4 5 ○○○○○ HUNGER SCALE								
Mid-morning ○○○○○								
Lunch 1 2 3 4 5 ○○○○○ HUNGER SCALE								
Mid-afternoon ○○○○○								
Dinner 1 2 3 4 5 ○○○○○ HUNGER SCALE								
Evening ○○○○○								

Coffees/teas [ ]   Fluid intake ⊔⊔⊔⊔⊔⊔⊔⊔⊔⊔   Daily totals

SUNDAY

	Time		Quantity	Fat	Protein	Carbs	Fibre	kJ/Cal
Breakfast 1 2 3 4 5 ○○○○○ HUNGER SCALE								
Mid-morning ○○○○○								
Lunch 1 2 3 4 5 ○○○○○ HUNGER SCALE								
Mid-afternoon ○○○○○								
Dinner 1 2 3 4 5 ○○○○○ HUNGER SCALE								
Evening ○○○○○								

Coffees/teas [ ]   Fluid intake ⊔⊔⊔⊔⊔⊔⊔⊔⊔⊔   Daily totals

Units of alcohol this week [ ]   Total alcohol kJ/Cal [ ]

Vitamins and supplements

WEEKLY TOTALS	Fat	Protein	Carbs	Fibre	kJ/Cal

WEEKLY PERSONAL SUMMARY

Mood 1 2 3 4 5 ○○○○○   **Appetite** 1 2 3 4 5 ○○○○○

Energy level 1 2 3 4 5 ○○○○○   **Stress level** 1 2 3 4 5 ○○○○○

Hours of sleep [ ]   **Sleep quality** 1 2 3 4 5 ○○○○○

kJ/Cal intake

Planned kJ/Cal	
Actual kJ/Cal	

Difference [+/-]

Weight at end of week

BMI at end of week

Injuries or illnesses

160

EXERCISE DIARY

STRENGTH TRAINING

Exercise	Focus area	SET 1		SET 2		SET 3		SET4		Equipment	Ease
		Reps	Weight	Reps	Weight	Reps	Weight	Reps	Weight		

CARDIO TRAINING

Exercise	Time	Distance	Intensity	Heart rate	Ease	kJ/Cal burnt

Total kJ/Cal burnt

INCIDENTAL EXERCISE

Day	Activity	Day	Activity

WEEK BEGINNING / /

Weight at start of week

BMI at start of week

Planned kJ/Cal this week

Possible diet-busting occasions this week

Planned exercise sessions this week

	Exercise	Completed [Y/N]
Monday		
Tuesday		
Wednesday		
Thursday		
Friday		
Saturday		
Sunday		

FOOD DIARY

MONDAY

	Time		Quantity	Fat	Protein	Carbs	Fibre	kJ/Cal
Breakfast 1 2 3 4 5 ○○○○○ HUNGER SCALE								
Mid-morning ○○○○○								
Lunch 1 2 3 4 5 ○○○○○ HUNGER SCALE								
Mid-afternoon ○○○○○								
Dinner 1 2 3 4 5 ○○○○○ HUNGER SCALE								
Evening ○○○○○								

Coffees/teas _____ Fluid intake ▽▽▽▽▽▽▽▽▽▽ Daily totals

TUESDAY

	Time		Quantity	Fat	Protein	Carbs	Fibre	kJ/Cal
Breakfast 1 2 3 4 5 ○○○○○ HUNGER SCALE								
Mid-morning ○○○○○								
Lunch 1 2 3 4 5 ○○○○○ HUNGER SCALE								
Mid-afternoon ○○○○○								
Dinner 1 2 3 4 5 ○○○○○ HUNGER SCALE								
Evening ○○○○○								

Coffees/teas _____ Fluid intake ▽▽▽▽▽▽▽▽▽▽ Daily totals

WEDNESDAY

	Time		Quantity	Fat	Protein	Carbs	Fibre	kJ/Cal
Breakfast 1 2 3 4 5 ○ ○ ○ ○ ○ HUNGER SCALE								
Mid-morning ○ ○ ○ ○ ○								
Lunch 1 2 3 4 5 ○ ○ ○ ○ ○ HUNGER SCALE								
Mid-afternoon ○ ○ ○ ○ ○								
Dinner 1 2 3 4 5 ○ ○ ○ ○ ○ HUNGER SCALE								
Evening ○ ○ ○ ○ ○								

Coffees/teas   Fluid intake ▽▽▽▽▽▽▽▽▽▽   Daily totals

THURSDAY

	Time		Quantity	Fat	Protein	Carbs	Fibre	kJ/Cal
Breakfast 1 2 3 4 5 ○ ○ ○ ○ ○ HUNGER SCALE								
Mid-morning ○ ○ ○ ○ ○								
Lunch 1 2 3 4 5 ○ ○ ○ ○ ○ HUNGER SCALE								
Mid-afternoon ○ ○ ○ ○ ○								
Dinner 1 2 3 4 5 ○ ○ ○ ○ ○ HUNGER SCALE								
Evening ○ ○ ○ ○ ○								

Coffees/teas   Fluid intake ▽▽▽▽▽▽▽▽▽▽   Daily totals

FRIDAY

	Time		Quantity	Fat	Protein	Carbs	Fibre	kJ/Cal
Breakfast 1 2 3 4 5 ○ ○ ○ ○ ○ HUNGER SCALE								
Mid-morning ○ ○ ○ ○ ○								
Lunch 1 2 3 4 5 ○ ○ ○ ○ ○ HUNGER SCALE								
Mid-afternoon ○ ○ ○ ○ ○								
Dinner 1 2 3 4 5 ○ ○ ○ ○ ○ HUNGER SCALE								
Evening ○ ○ ○ ○ ○								

Coffees/teas   Fluid intake ▽▽▽▽▽▽▽▽▽▽   Daily totals

SATURDAY

	Time		Quantity	Fat	Protein	Carbs	Fibre	kJ/Cal
Breakfast 1 2 3 4 5 ○ ○ ○ ○ ○ HUNGER SCALE								
Mid-morning ○ ○ ○ ○ ○								
Lunch 1 2 3 4 5 ○ ○ ○ ○ ○ HUNGER SCALE								
Mid-afternoon ○ ○ ○ ○ ○								
Dinner 1 2 3 4 5 ○ ○ ○ ○ ○ HUNGER SCALE								
Evening ○ ○ ○ ○ ○								

Coffees/teas   Fluid intake ▽▽▽▽▽▽▽▽▽▽   Daily totals

SUNDAY

	Time		Quantity	Fat	Protein	Carbs	Fibre	kJ/Cal
Breakfast 1 2 3 4 5 ○ ○ ○ ○ ○ HUNGER SCALE								
Mid-morning ○ ○ ○ ○ ○								
Lunch 1 2 3 4 5 ○ ○ ○ ○ ○ HUNGER SCALE								
Mid-afternoon ○ ○ ○ ○ ○								
Dinner 1 2 3 4 5 ○ ○ ○ ○ ○ HUNGER SCALE								
Evening ○ ○ ○ ○ ○								

Coffees/teas   Fluid intake ▽▽▽▽▽▽▽▽▽▽   Daily totals

Units of alcohol this week   **Total alcohol kJ/Cal**

Vitamins and supplements

WEEKLY TOTALS	Fat	Protein	Carbs	Fibre	kJ/Cal

WEEKLY PERSONAL SUMMARY

Mood 1 2 3 4 5 ○ ○ ○ ○ ○   **Appetite** 1 2 3 4 5 ○ ○ ○ ○ ○

Energy level 1 2 3 4 5 ○ ○ ○ ○ ○   **Stress level** 1 2 3 4 5 ○ ○ ○ ○ ○

Hours of sleep   **Sleep quality** 1 2 3 4 5 ○ ○ ○ ○ ○

kJ/Cal intake

Planned kJ/Cal	
Actual kJ/Cal	
Difference [+/-]	

Weight at end of week

BMI at end of week

Injuries or illnesses

EXERCISE DIARY

STRENGTH TRAINING		SET 1		SET 2		SET 3		SET 4			
Exercise	Focus area	Reps	Weight	Reps	Weight	Reps	Weight	Reps	Weight	Equipment	Ease

CARDIO TRAINING

Exercise	Time	Distance	Intensity	Heart rate	Ease	kJ/Cal burnt

Total kJ/Cal burnt

INCIDENTAL EXERCISE

Day	Activity	Day	Activity

WEEK BEGINNING   /   /

Weight at start of week

BMI at start of week

Planned kJ/Cal this week

Possible diet-busting occasions this week

Planned exercise sessions this week

	Exercise	Completed [Y/N]
Monday		
Tuesday		
Wednesday		
Thursday		
Friday		
Saturday		
Sunday		

FOOD DIARY

MONDAY

	Time		Quantity	Fat	Protein	Carbs	Fibre	kJ/Cal
Breakfast 1 2 3 4 5 ○ ○ ○ ○ ○ HUNGER SCALE								
Mid-morning ○ ○ ○ ○ ○								
Lunch 1 2 3 4 5 ○ ○ ○ ○ ○ HUNGER SCALE								
Mid-afternoon ○ ○ ○ ○ ○								
Dinner 1 2 3 4 5 ○ ○ ○ ○ ○ HUNGER SCALE								
Evening ○ ○ ○ ○ ○								

Coffees/teas   Fluid intake ▽▽▽▽▽▽▽▽▽▽   Daily totals

TUESDAY

	Time		Quantity	Fat	Protein	Carbs	Fibre	kJ/Cal
Breakfast 1 2 3 4 5 ○ ○ ○ ○ ○ HUNGER SCALE								
Mid-morning ○ ○ ○ ○ ○								
Lunch 1 2 3 4 5 ○ ○ ○ ○ ○ HUNGER SCALE								
Mid-afternoon ○ ○ ○ ○ ○								
Dinner 1 2 3 4 5 ○ ○ ○ ○ ○ HUNGER SCALE								
Evening ○ ○ ○ ○ ○								

Coffees/teas   Fluid intake ▽▽▽▽▽▽▽▽▽▽   Daily totals

WEDNESDAY

	Time		Quantity	Fat	Protein	Carbs	Fibre	kJ/Cal
Breakfast 1 2 3 4 5 ○ ○ ○ ○ ○ HUNGER SCALE								
Mid-morning ○ ○ ○ ○ ○								
Lunch 1 2 3 4 5 ○ ○ ○ ○ ○ HUNGER SCALE								
Mid-afternoon ○ ○ ○ ○ ○								
Dinner 1 2 3 4 5 ○ ○ ○ ○ ○ HUNGER SCALE								
Evening ○ ○ ○ ○ ○								

Coffees/teas   Fluid intake ⊔ ⊔ ⊔ ⊔ ⊔ ⊔ ⊔ ⊔ ⊔ ⊔   Daily totals

THURSDAY

	Time		Quantity	Fat	Protein	Carbs	Fibre	kJ/Cal
Breakfast 1 2 3 4 5 ○ ○ ○ ○ ○ HUNGER SCALE								
Mid-morning ○ ○ ○ ○ ○								
Lunch 1 2 3 4 5 ○ ○ ○ ○ ○ HUNGER SCALE								
Mid-afternoon ○ ○ ○ ○ ○								
Dinner 1 2 3 4 5 ○ ○ ○ ○ ○ HUNGER SCALE								
Evening ○ ○ ○ ○ ○								

Coffees/teas   Fluid intake ⊔ ⊔ ⊔ ⊔ ⊔ ⊔ ⊔ ⊔ ⊔ ⊔   Daily totals

FRIDAY

	Time		Quantity	Fat	Protein	Carbs	Fibre	kJ/Cal
Breakfast 1 2 3 4 5 ○ ○ ○ ○ ○ HUNGER SCALE								
Mid-morning ○ ○ ○ ○ ○								
Lunch 1 2 3 4 5 ○ ○ ○ ○ ○ HUNGER SCALE								
Mid-afternoon ○ ○ ○ ○ ○								
Dinner 1 2 3 4 5 ○ ○ ○ ○ ○ HUNGER SCALE								
Evening ○ ○ ○ ○ ○								

Coffees/teas   Fluid intake ⊔ ⊔ ⊔ ⊔ ⊔ ⊔ ⊔ ⊔ ⊔ ⊔   Daily totals

SATURDAY

	Time		Quantity	Fat	Protein	Carbs	Fibre	kJ/Cal
Breakfast 1 2 3 4 5 ○○○○○ HUNGER SCALE								
Mid-morning ○○○○○								
Lunch 1 2 3 4 5 ○○○○○ HUNGER SCALE								
Mid-afternoon ○○○○○								
Dinner 1 2 3 4 5 ○○○○○ HUNGER SCALE								
Evening ○○○○○								

Coffees/teas ☐ Fluid intake ▽▽▽▽▽▽▽▽▽▽ Daily totals

SUNDAY

	Time		Quantity	Fat	Protein	Carbs	Fibre	kJ/Cal
Breakfast 1 2 3 4 5 ○○○○○ HUNGER SCALE								
Mid-morning ○○○○○								
Lunch 1 2 3 4 5 ○○○○○ HUNGER SCALE								
Mid-afternoon ○○○○○								
Dinner 1 2 3 4 5 ○○○○○ HUNGER SCALE								
Evening ○○○○○								

Coffees/teas ☐ Fluid intake ▽▽▽▽▽▽▽▽▽▽ Daily totals

Units of alcohol this week ☐   Total alcohol kJ/Cal ☐

Vitamins and supplements

WEEKLY TOTALS	Fat	Protein	Carbs	Fibre	kJ/Cal

WEEKLY PERSONAL SUMMARY

Mood 1 2 3 4 5 ○○○○○   **Appetite** 1 2 3 4 5 ○○○○○

Energy level 1 2 3 4 5 ○○○○○   **Stress level** 1 2 3 4 5 ○○○○○

Hours of sleep ☐   **Sleep quality** 1 2 3 4 5 ○○○○○

kJ/Cal intake

Planned kJ/Cal	
Actual kJ/Cal	
Difference [+/-]	

Weight at end of week

BMI at end of week

Injuries or illnesses

EXERCISE DIARY

STRENGTH TRAINING		SET 1		SET 2		SET 3		SET4			
Exercise	Focus area	Reps	Weight	Reps	Weight	Reps	Weight	Reps	Weight	Equipment	Ease

CARDIO TRAINING

Exercise	Time	Distance	Intensity	Heart rate	Ease	kJ/Cal burnt

Total kJ/Cal burnt

INCIDENTAL EXERCISE

Day	Activity	Day	Activity

WEEK BEGINNING   /   /

Weight at start of week

BMI at start of week

Planned kJ/Cal this week

Possible diet-busting occasions this week

Planned exercise sessions this week

	Exercise	Completed [Y/N]
Monday		
Tuesday		
Wednesday		
Thursday		
Friday		
Saturday		
Sunday		

FOOD DIARY

MONDAY

	Time				Quantity	Fat	Protein	Carbs	Fibre	kJ/Cal
Breakfast 1 2 3 4 5 ○○○○○ HUNGER SCALE										
Mid-morning ○○○○○										
Lunch 1 2 3 4 5 ○○○○○ HUNGER SCALE										
Mid-afternoon ○○○○○										
Dinner 1 2 3 4 5 ○○○○○ HUNGER SCALE										
Evening ○○○○○										

Coffees/teas   Fluid intake ▽▽▽▽▽▽▽▽▽▽   Daily totals

TUESDAY

	Time				Quantity	Fat	Protein	Carbs	Fibre	kJ/Cal
Breakfast 1 2 3 4 5 ○○○○○ HUNGER SCALE										
Mid-morning ○○○○○										
Lunch 1 2 3 4 5 ○○○○○ HUNGER SCALE										
Mid-afternoon ○○○○○										
Dinner 1 2 3 4 5 ○○○○○ HUNGER SCALE										
Evening ○○○○○										

Coffees/teas   Fluid intake ▽▽▽▽▽▽▽▽▽▽   Daily totals

WEDNESDAY

	Time		Quantity	Fat	Protein	Carbs	Fibre	kJ/Cal
Breakfast 1 2 3 4 5 ○ ○ ○ ○ ○ HUNGER SCALE								
Mid-morning ○ ○ ○ ○ ○								
Lunch 1 2 3 4 5 ○ ○ ○ ○ ○ HUNGER SCALE								
Mid-afternoon ○ ○ ○ ○ ○								
Dinner 1 2 3 4 5 ○ ○ ○ ○ ○ HUNGER SCALE								
Evening ○ ○ ○ ○ ○								

Coffees/teas | Fluid intake ▽▽▽▽▽▽▽▽▽▽ | Daily totals

THURSDAY

	Time		Quantity	Fat	Protein	Carbs	Fibre	kJ/Cal
Breakfast 1 2 3 4 5 ○ ○ ○ ○ ○ HUNGER SCALE								
Mid-morning ○ ○ ○ ○ ○								
Lunch 1 2 3 4 5 ○ ○ ○ ○ ○ HUNGER SCALE								
Mid-afternoon ○ ○ ○ ○ ○								
Dinner 1 2 3 4 5 ○ ○ ○ ○ ○ HUNGER SCALE								
Evening ○ ○ ○ ○ ○								

Coffees/teas | Fluid intake ▽▽▽▽▽▽▽▽▽▽ | Daily totals

FRIDAY

	Time		Quantity	Fat	Protein	Carbs	Fibre	kJ/Cal
Breakfast 1 2 3 4 5 ○ ○ ○ ○ ○ HUNGER SCALE								
Mid-morning ○ ○ ○ ○ ○								
Lunch 1 2 3 4 5 ○ ○ ○ ○ ○ HUNGER SCALE								
Mid-afternoon ○ ○ ○ ○ ○								
Dinner 1 2 3 4 5 ○ ○ ○ ○ ○ HUNGER SCALE								
Evening ○ ○ ○ ○ ○								

Coffees/teas | Fluid intake ▽▽▽▽▽▽▽▽▽▽ | Daily totals

SATURDAY

	Time		Quantity	Fat	Protein	Carbs	Fibre	kJ/Cal
Breakfast 1 2 3 4 5 ○ ○ ○ ○ ○ HUNGER SCALE								
Mid-morning ○ ○ ○ ○ ○								
Lunch 1 2 3 4 5 ○ ○ ○ ○ ○ HUNGER SCALE								
Mid-afternoon ○ ○ ○ ○ ○								
Dinner 1 2 3 4 5 ○ ○ ○ ○ ○ HUNGER SCALE								
Evening ○ ○ ○ ○ ○								

Coffees/teas ☐ Fluid intake ☐☐☐☐☐☐☐☐☐☐ Daily totals

SUNDAY

	Time		Quantity	Fat	Protein	Carbs	Fibre	kJ/Cal
Breakfast 1 2 3 4 5 ○ ○ ○ ○ ○ HUNGER SCALE								
Mid-morning ○ ○ ○ ○ ○								
Lunch 1 2 3 4 5 ○ ○ ○ ○ ○ HUNGER SCALE								
Mid-afternoon ○ ○ ○ ○ ○								
Dinner 1 2 3 4 5 ○ ○ ○ ○ ○ HUNGER SCALE								
Evening ○ ○ ○ ○ ○								

Coffees/teas ☐ Fluid intake ☐☐☐☐☐☐☐☐☐☐ Daily totals

Units of alcohol this week ☐   Total alcohol kJ/Cal ☐

Vitamins and supplements

WEEKLY TOTALS	Fat	Protein	Carbs	Fibre	kJ/Cal

WEEKLY PERSONAL SUMMARY

Mood 1 2 3 4 5 ○ ○ ○ ○ ○   **Appetite** 1 2 3 4 5 ○ ○ ○ ○ ○

Energy level 1 2 3 4 5 ○ ○ ○ ○ ○   **Stress level** 1 2 3 4 5 ○ ○ ○ ○ ○

Hours of sleep ☐   **Sleep quality** 1 2 3 4 5 ○ ○ ○ ○ ○

Injuries or illnesses

kJ/Cal intake

Planned kJ/Cal	
Actual kJ/Cal	
Difference [+/-]	

Weight at end of week

BMI at end of week

EXERCISE DIARY

STRENGTH TRAINING		SET 1		SET 2		SET 3		SET4			
Exercise	Focus area	Reps	Weight	Reps	Weight	Reps	Weight	Reps	Weight	Equipment	Ease

CARDIO TRAINING

Exercise	Time	Distance	Intensity	Heart rate	Ease	kJ/Cal burnt

Total kJ/Cal burnt

INCIDENTAL EXERCISE

Day	Activity	Day	Activity

WEEK BEGINNING   /   /

Weight at start of week

BMI at start of week

Planned kJ/Cal this week

Possible diet-busting occasions this week

Planned exercise sessions this week

	Exercise	Completed [Y/N]
Monday		
Tuesday		
Wednesday		
Thursday		
Friday		
Saturday		
Sunday		

FOOD DIARY

MONDAY

	Time		Quantity	Fat	Protein	Carbs	Fibre	kJ/Cal
Breakfast 1 2 3 4 5 ○○○○○ HUNGER SCALE								
Mid-morning ○○○○○								
Lunch 1 2 3 4 5 ○○○○○ HUNGER SCALE								
Mid-afternoon ○○○○○								
Dinner 1 2 3 4 5 ○○○○○ HUNGER SCALE								
Evening ○○○○○								

Coffees/teas   Fluid intake ▽▽▽▽▽▽▽▽▽▽   Daily totals

TUESDAY

	Time		Quantity	Fat	Protein	Carbs	Fibre	kJ/Cal
Breakfast 1 2 3 4 5 ○○○○○ HUNGER SCALE								
Mid-morning ○○○○○								
Lunch 1 2 3 4 5 ○○○○○ HUNGER SCALE								
Mid-afternoon ○○○○○								
Dinner 1 2 3 4 5 ○○○○○ HUNGER SCALE								
Evening ○○○○○								

Coffees/teas   Fluid intake ▽▽▽▽▽▽▽▽▽▽   Daily totals

WEDNESDAY

	Time		Quantity	Fat	Protein	Carbs	Fibre	kJ/Cal
Breakfast 1 2 3 4 5 ○ ○ ○ ○ ○ HUNGER SCALE								
Mid-morning ○ ○ ○ ○ ○								
Lunch 1 2 3 4 5 ○ ○ ○ ○ ○ HUNGER SCALE								
Mid-afternoon ○ ○ ○ ○ ○								
Dinner 1 2 3 4 5 ○ ○ ○ ○ ○ HUNGER SCALE								
Evening ○ ○ ○ ○ ○								
Coffees/teas	Fluid intake ⊔⊔⊔⊔⊔⊔⊔⊔⊔⊔	Daily totals						

THURSDAY

	Time		Quantity	Fat	Protein	Carbs	Fibre	kJ/Cal
Breakfast 1 2 3 4 5 ○ ○ ○ ○ ○ HUNGER SCALE								
Mid-morning ○ ○ ○ ○ ○								
Lunch 1 2 3 4 5 ○ ○ ○ ○ ○ HUNGER SCALE								
Mid-afternoon ○ ○ ○ ○ ○								
Dinner 1 2 3 4 5 ○ ○ ○ ○ ○ HUNGER SCALE								
Evening ○ ○ ○ ○ ○								
Coffees/teas	Fluid intake ⊔⊔⊔⊔⊔⊔⊔⊔⊔⊔	Daily totals						

FRIDAY

	Time		Quantity	Fat	Protein	Carbs	Fibre	kJ/Cal
Breakfast 1 2 3 4 5 ○ ○ ○ ○ ○ HUNGER SCALE								
Mid-morning ○ ○ ○ ○ ○								
Lunch 1 2 3 4 5 ○ ○ ○ ○ ○ HUNGER SCALE								
Mid-afternoon ○ ○ ○ ○ ○								
Dinner 1 2 3 4 5 ○ ○ ○ ○ ○ HUNGER SCALE								
Evening ○ ○ ○ ○ ○								
Coffees/teas	Fluid intake ⊔⊔⊔⊔⊔⊔⊔⊔⊔⊔	Daily totals						

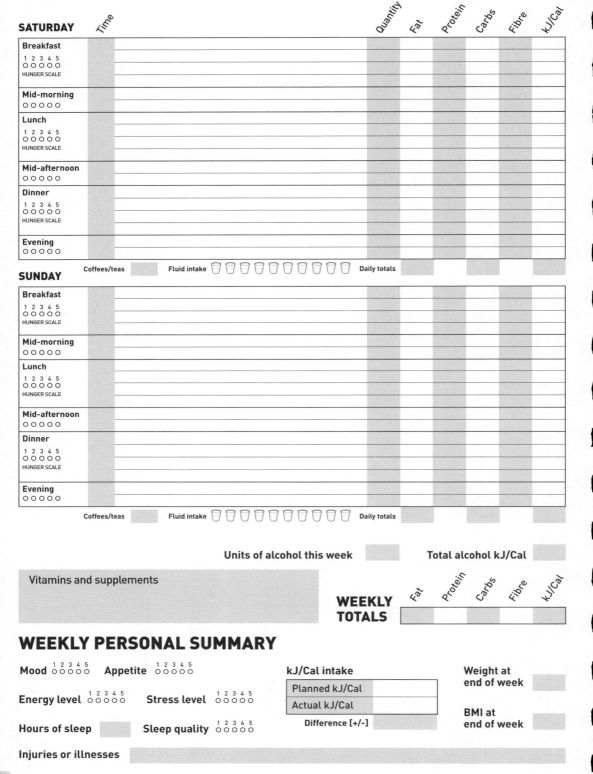

SATURDAY

	Time		Quantity	Fat	Protein	Carbs	Fibre	kJ/Cal
Breakfast 1 2 3 4 5 ○○○○○ HUNGER SCALE								
Mid-morning ○○○○○								
Lunch 1 2 3 4 5 ○○○○○ HUNGER SCALE								
Mid-afternoon ○○○○○								
Dinner 1 2 3 4 5 ○○○○○ HUNGER SCALE								
Evening ○○○○○								

Coffees/teas   Fluid intake ⊔⊔⊔⊔⊔⊔⊔⊔⊔⊔   Daily totals

SUNDAY

	Time		Quantity	Fat	Protein	Carbs	Fibre	kJ/Cal
Breakfast 1 2 3 4 5 ○○○○○ HUNGER SCALE								
Mid-morning ○○○○○								
Lunch 1 2 3 4 5 ○○○○○ HUNGER SCALE								
Mid-afternoon ○○○○○								
Dinner 1 2 3 4 5 ○○○○○ HUNGER SCALE								
Evening ○○○○○								

Coffees/teas   Fluid intake ⊔⊔⊔⊔⊔⊔⊔⊔⊔⊔   Daily totals

Units of alcohol this week   Total alcohol kJ/Cal

Vitamins and supplements

WEEKLY TOTALS	Fat	Protein	Carbs	Fibre	kJ/Cal

WEEKLY PERSONAL SUMMARY

Mood 1 2 3 4 5 ○○○○○   **Appetite** 1 2 3 4 5 ○○○○○

Energy level 1 2 3 4 5 ○○○○○   **Stress level** 1 2 3 4 5 ○○○○○

Hours of sleep   **Sleep quality** 1 2 3 4 5 ○○○○○

Injuries or illnesses

kJ/Cal intake

Planned kJ/Cal	
Actual kJ/Cal	

Difference [+/-]

Weight at end of week

BMI at end of week

EXERCISE DIARY

STRENGTH TRAINING		SET 1		SET 2		SET 3		SET4			
Exercise	Focus area	Reps	Weight	Reps	Weight	Reps	Weight	Reps	Weight	Equipment	Ease

CARDIO TRAINING

Exercise	Time	Distance	Intensity	Heart rate	Ease	kJ/Cal burnt

Total kJ/Cal burnt

INCIDENTAL EXERCISE

Day	Activity	Day	Activity

WEEK BEGINNING   /   /

Weight at start of week

BMI at start of week

Planned kJ/Cal this week

Possible diet-busting occasions this week

Planned exercise sessions this week

	Exercise	Completed [Y/N]
Monday		
Tuesday		
Wednesday		
Thursday		
Friday		
Saturday		
Sunday		

FOOD DIARY

MONDAY

	Time							Quantity	Fat	Protein	Carbs	Fibre	kJ/Cal
Breakfast 1 2 3 4 5 ○○○○○ HUNGER SCALE													
Mid-morning ○○○○○													
Lunch 1 2 3 4 5 ○○○○○ HUNGER SCALE													
Mid-afternoon ○○○○○													
Dinner 1 2 3 4 5 ○○○○○ HUNGER SCALE													
Evening ○○○○○													

Coffees/teas   Fluid intake ☐☐☐☐☐☐☐☐☐☐   Daily totals

TUESDAY

Breakfast 1 2 3 4 5 ○○○○○ HUNGER SCALE													
Mid-morning ○○○○○													
Lunch 1 2 3 4 5 ○○○○○ HUNGER SCALE													
Mid-afternoon ○○○○○													
Dinner 1 2 3 4 5 ○○○○○ HUNGER SCALE													
Evening ○○○○○													

Coffees/teas   Fluid intake ☐☐☐☐☐☐☐☐☐☐   Daily totals

WEDNESDAY

	Time		Quantity	Fat	Protein	Carbs	Fibre	kJ/Cal
Breakfast 1 2 3 4 5 ○○○○○ HUNGER SCALE								
Mid-morning ○○○○○								
Lunch 1 2 3 4 5 ○○○○○ HUNGER SCALE								
Mid-afternoon ○○○○○								
Dinner 1 2 3 4 5 ○○○○○ HUNGER SCALE								
Evening ○○○○○								

Coffees/teas   **Fluid intake** ⊔⊔⊔⊔⊔⊔⊔⊔⊔⊔   **Daily totals**

THURSDAY

	Time		Quantity	Fat	Protein	Carbs	Fibre	kJ/Cal
Breakfast 1 2 3 4 5 ○○○○○ HUNGER SCALE								
Mid-morning ○○○○○								
Lunch 1 2 3 4 5 ○○○○○ HUNGER SCALE								
Mid-afternoon ○○○○○								
Dinner 1 2 3 4 5 ○○○○○ HUNGER SCALE								
Evening ○○○○○								

Coffees/teas   **Fluid intake** ⊔⊔⊔⊔⊔⊔⊔⊔⊔⊔   **Daily totals**

FRIDAY

	Time		Quantity	Fat	Protein	Carbs	Fibre	kJ/Cal
Breakfast 1 2 3 4 5 ○○○○○ HUNGER SCALE								
Mid-morning ○○○○○								
Lunch 1 2 3 4 5 ○○○○○ HUNGER SCALE								
Mid-afternoon ○○○○○								
Dinner 1 2 3 4 5 ○○○○○ HUNGER SCALE								
Evening ○○○○○								

Coffees/teas   **Fluid intake** ⊔⊔⊔⊔⊔⊔⊔⊔⊔⊔   **Daily totals**

SATURDAY

	Time		Quantity	Fat	Protein	Carbs	Fibre	kJ/Cal
Breakfast 1 2 3 4 5 ○ ○ ○ ○ ○ HUNGER SCALE								
Mid-morning ○ ○ ○ ○ ○								
Lunch 1 2 3 4 5 ○ ○ ○ ○ ○ HUNGER SCALE								
Mid-afternoon ○ ○ ○ ○ ○								
Dinner 1 2 3 4 5 ○ ○ ○ ○ ○ HUNGER SCALE								
Evening ○ ○ ○ ○ ○								

Coffees/teas   Fluid intake ⬜⬜⬜⬜⬜⬜⬜⬜⬜⬜   Daily totals

SUNDAY

	Time		Quantity	Fat	Protein	Carbs	Fibre	kJ/Cal
Breakfast 1 2 3 4 5 ○ ○ ○ ○ ○ HUNGER SCALE								
Mid-morning ○ ○ ○ ○ ○								
Lunch 1 2 3 4 5 ○ ○ ○ ○ ○ HUNGER SCALE								
Mid-afternoon ○ ○ ○ ○ ○								
Dinner 1 2 3 4 5 ○ ○ ○ ○ ○ HUNGER SCALE								
Evening ○ ○ ○ ○ ○								

Coffees/teas   Fluid intake ⬜⬜⬜⬜⬜⬜⬜⬜⬜⬜   Daily totals

Units of alcohol this week   **Total alcohol kJ/Cal**

Vitamins and supplements

WEEKLY TOTALS	Fat	Protein	Carbs	Fibre	kJ/Cal

WEEKLY PERSONAL SUMMARY

Mood 1 2 3 4 5 ○ ○ ○ ○ ○   **Appetite** 1 2 3 4 5 ○ ○ ○ ○ ○

Energy level 1 2 3 4 5 ○ ○ ○ ○ ○   **Stress level** 1 2 3 4 5 ○ ○ ○ ○ ○

Hours of sleep   **Sleep quality** 1 2 3 4 5 ○ ○ ○ ○ ○

Injuries or illnesses

kJ/Cal intake	
Planned kJ/Cal	
Actual kJ/Cal	
Difference [+/-]	

Weight at end of week

BMI at end of week

EXERCISE DIARY

STRENGTH TRAINING		SET 1		SET 2		SET 3		SET4			
Exercise	Focus area	Reps	Weight	Reps	Weight	Reps	Weight	Reps	Weight	Equipment	Ease

CARDIO TRAINING

Exercise	Time	Distance	Intensity	Heart rate	Ease	kJ/Cal burnt

Total kJ/Cal burnt

INCIDENTAL EXERCISE

Day	Activity	Day	Activity

WEEK BEGINNING ☐ / ☐ / ☐

Weight at start of week ☐

BMI at start of week ☐

Planned kJ/Cal this week ☐

Possible diet-busting occasions this week

Planned exercise sessions this week

	Exercise	Completed [Y/N]
Monday		
Tuesday		
Wednesday		
Thursday		
Friday		
Saturday		
Sunday		

FOOD DIARY

MONDAY

	Time		Quantity	Fat	Protein	Carbs	Fibre	kJ/Cal
Breakfast 1 2 3 4 5 ○○○○○ HUNGER SCALE								
Mid-morning ○○○○○								
Lunch 1 2 3 4 5 ○○○○○ HUNGER SCALE								
Mid-afternoon ○○○○○								
Dinner 1 2 3 4 5 ○○○○○ HUNGER SCALE								
Evening ○○○○○								

Coffees/teas ☐   Fluid intake ▽▽▽▽▽▽▽▽▽▽   Daily totals

TUESDAY

	Time		Quantity	Fat	Protein	Carbs	Fibre	kJ/Cal
Breakfast 1 2 3 4 5 ○○○○○ HUNGER SCALE								
Mid-morning ○○○○○								
Lunch 1 2 3 4 5 ○○○○○ HUNGER SCALE								
Mid-afternoon ○○○○○								
Dinner 1 2 3 4 5 ○○○○○ HUNGER SCALE								
Evening ○○○○○								

Coffees/teas ☐   Fluid intake ▽▽▽▽▽▽▽▽▽▽   Daily totals

WEDNESDAY

	Time		Quantity	Fat	Protein	Carbs	Fibre	kJ/Cal
Breakfast 1 2 3 4 5 ○○○○○ HUNGER SCALE								
Mid-morning ○○○○○								
Lunch 1 2 3 4 5 ○○○○○ HUNGER SCALE								
Mid-afternoon ○○○○○								
Dinner 1 2 3 4 5 ○○○○○ HUNGER SCALE								
Evening ○○○○○								

Coffees/teas   Fluid intake ▽▽▽▽▽▽▽▽▽▽   Daily totals

THURSDAY

	Time		Quantity	Fat	Protein	Carbs	Fibre	kJ/Cal
Breakfast 1 2 3 4 5 ○○○○○ HUNGER SCALE								
Mid-morning ○○○○○								
Lunch 1 2 3 4 5 ○○○○○ HUNGER SCALE								
Mid-afternoon ○○○○○								
Dinner 1 2 3 4 5 ○○○○○ HUNGER SCALE								
Evening ○○○○○								

Coffees/teas   Fluid intake ▽▽▽▽▽▽▽▽▽▽   Daily totals

FRIDAY

	Time		Quantity	Fat	Protein	Carbs	Fibre	kJ/Cal
Breakfast 1 2 3 4 5 ○○○○○ HUNGER SCALE								
Mid-morning ○○○○○								
Lunch 1 2 3 4 5 ○○○○○ HUNGER SCALE								
Mid-afternoon ○○○○○								
Dinner 1 2 3 4 5 ○○○○○ HUNGER SCALE								
Evening ○○○○○								

Coffees/teas   Fluid intake ▽▽▽▽▽▽▽▽▽▽   Daily totals

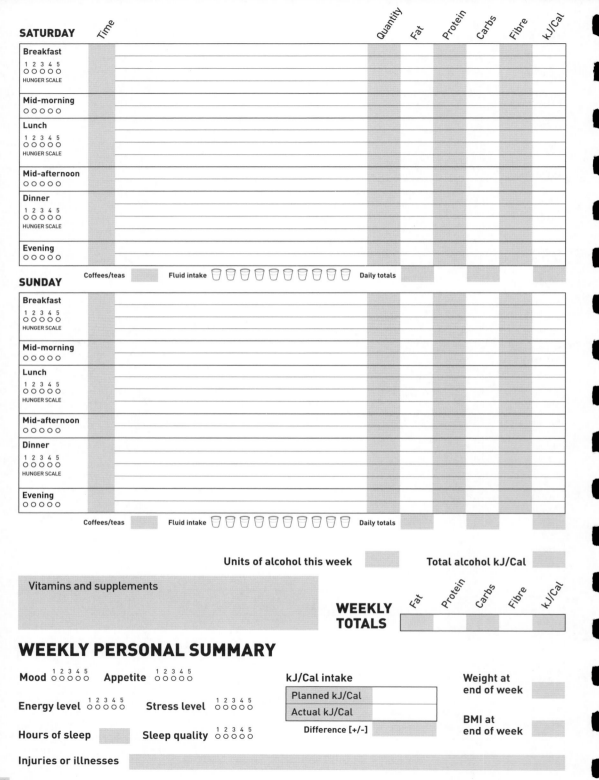

SATURDAY

	Time		Quantity	Fat	Protein	Carbs	Fibre	kJ/Cal
Breakfast 1 2 3 4 5 ○ ○ ○ ○ ○ HUNGER SCALE								
Mid-morning ○ ○ ○ ○ ○								
Lunch 1 2 3 4 5 ○ ○ ○ ○ ○ HUNGER SCALE								
Mid-afternoon ○ ○ ○ ○ ○								
Dinner 1 2 3 4 5 ○ ○ ○ ○ ○ HUNGER SCALE								
Evening ○ ○ ○ ○ ○								

Coffees/teas ▢   Fluid intake ▽▽▽▽▽▽▽▽▽▽   Daily totals

SUNDAY

	Time		Quantity	Fat	Protein	Carbs	Fibre	kJ/Cal
Breakfast 1 2 3 4 5 ○ ○ ○ ○ ○ HUNGER SCALE								
Mid-morning ○ ○ ○ ○ ○								
Lunch 1 2 3 4 5 ○ ○ ○ ○ ○ HUNGER SCALE								
Mid-afternoon ○ ○ ○ ○ ○								
Dinner 1 2 3 4 5 ○ ○ ○ ○ ○ HUNGER SCALE								
Evening ○ ○ ○ ○ ○								

Coffees/teas ▢   Fluid intake ▽▽▽▽▽▽▽▽▽▽   Daily totals

Units of alcohol this week ▢   Total alcohol kJ/Cal

Vitamins and supplements

WEEKLY TOTALS	Fat	Protein	Carbs	Fibre	kJ/Cal

WEEKLY PERSONAL SUMMARY

Mood 1 2 3 4 5 ○ ○ ○ ○ ○   **Appetite** 1 2 3 4 5 ○ ○ ○ ○ ○

Energy level 1 2 3 4 5 ○ ○ ○ ○ ○   **Stress level** 1 2 3 4 5 ○ ○ ○ ○ ○

Hours of sleep ▢   **Sleep quality** 1 2 3 4 5 ○ ○ ○ ○ ○

kJ/Cal intake

Planned kJ/Cal	
Actual kJ/Cal	

Difference [+/-]

Weight at end of week

BMI at end of week

Injuries or illnesses

184

EXERCISE DIARY

STRENGTH TRAINING		SET 1		SET 2		SET 3		SET 4			
Exercise	Focus area	Reps	Weight	Reps	Weight	Reps	Weight	Reps	Weight	Equipment	Ease

CARDIO TRAINING

Exercise	Time	Distance	Intensity	Heart rate	Ease	kJ/Cal burnt

Total kJ/Cal burnt

INCIDENTAL EXERCISE

Day	Activity	Day	Activity

WEEK BEGINNING ___ / ___ / ___

Weight at start of week ▢

BMI at start of week ▢

Planned kJ/Cal this week ▢

Possible diet-busting occasions this week

▢

Planned exercise sessions this week

	Exercise	Completed [Y/N]
Monday		
Tuesday		
Wednesday		
Thursday		
Friday		
Saturday		
Sunday		

FOOD DIARY

MONDAY

Time		Quantity	Fat	Protein	Carbs	Fibre	kJ/Cal
Breakfast 1 2 3 4 5 ○○○○○ HUNGER SCALE							
Mid-morning ○○○○○							
Lunch 1 2 3 4 5 ○○○○○ HUNGER SCALE							
Mid-afternoon ○○○○○							
Dinner 1 2 3 4 5 ○○○○○ HUNGER SCALE							
Evening ○○○○○							

Coffees/teas ▢ Fluid intake ▽▽▽▽▽▽▽▽▽▽ Daily totals

TUESDAY

Time		Quantity	Fat	Protein	Carbs	Fibre	kJ/Cal
Breakfast 1 2 3 4 5 ○○○○○ HUNGER SCALE							
Mid-morning ○○○○○							
Lunch 1 2 3 4 5 ○○○○○ HUNGER SCALE							
Mid-afternoon ○○○○○							
Dinner 1 2 3 4 5 ○○○○○ HUNGER SCALE							
Evening ○○○○○							

Coffees/teas ▢ Fluid intake ▽▽▽▽▽▽▽▽▽▽ Daily totals

WEDNESDAY

	Time		Quantity	Fat	Protein	Carbs	Fibre	kJ/Cal
Breakfast 1 2 3 4 5 ○○○○○ HUNGER SCALE								
Mid-morning ○○○○○								
Lunch 1 2 3 4 5 ○○○○○ HUNGER SCALE								
Mid-afternoon ○○○○○								
Dinner 1 2 3 4 5 ○○○○○ HUNGER SCALE								
Evening ○○○○○								

Coffees/teas   Fluid intake ▽▽▽▽▽▽▽▽▽▽ Daily totals

THURSDAY

	Time		Quantity	Fat	Protein	Carbs	Fibre	kJ/Cal
Breakfast 1 2 3 4 5 ○○○○○ HUNGER SCALE								
Mid-morning ○○○○○								
Lunch 1 2 3 4 5 ○○○○○ HUNGER SCALE								
Mid-afternoon ○○○○○								
Dinner 1 2 3 4 5 ○○○○○ HUNGER SCALE								
Evening ○○○○○								

Coffees/teas   Fluid intake ▽▽▽▽▽▽▽▽▽▽ Daily totals

FRIDAY

	Time		Quantity	Fat	Protein	Carbs	Fibre	kJ/Cal
Breakfast 1 2 3 4 5 ○○○○○ HUNGER SCALE								
Mid-morning ○○○○○								
Lunch 1 2 3 4 5 ○○○○○ HUNGER SCALE								
Mid-afternoon ○○○○○								
Dinner 1 2 3 4 5 ○○○○○ HUNGER SCALE								
Evening ○○○○○								

Coffees/teas   Fluid intake ▽▽▽▽▽▽▽▽▽▽ Daily totals

SATURDAY

	Time		Quantity	Fat	Protein	Carbs	Fibre	kJ/Cal
Breakfast 1 2 3 4 5 ○ ○ ○ ○ ○ HUNGER SCALE								
Mid-morning ○ ○ ○ ○ ○								
Lunch 1 2 3 4 5 ○ ○ ○ ○ ○ HUNGER SCALE								
Mid-afternoon ○ ○ ○ ○ ○								
Dinner 1 2 3 4 5 ○ ○ ○ ○ ○ HUNGER SCALE								
Evening ○ ○ ○ ○ ○								

Coffees/teas ☐ Fluid intake 🥛🥛🥛🥛🥛🥛🥛🥛🥛🥛 Daily totals

SUNDAY

	Time		Quantity	Fat	Protein	Carbs	Fibre	kJ/Cal
Breakfast 1 2 3 4 5 ○ ○ ○ ○ ○ HUNGER SCALE								
Mid-morning ○ ○ ○ ○ ○								
Lunch 1 2 3 4 5 ○ ○ ○ ○ ○ HUNGER SCALE								
Mid-afternoon ○ ○ ○ ○ ○								
Dinner 1 2 3 4 5 ○ ○ ○ ○ ○ HUNGER SCALE								
Evening ○ ○ ○ ○ ○								

Coffees/teas ☐ Fluid intake 🥛🥛🥛🥛🥛🥛🥛🥛🥛🥛 Daily totals

Units of alcohol this week ☐   Total alcohol kJ/Cal ☐

Vitamins and supplements

	Fat	Protein	Carbs	Fibre	kJ/Cal
WEEKLY TOTALS					

WEEKLY PERSONAL SUMMARY

Mood 1 2 3 4 5 ○ ○ ○ ○ ○   **Appetite** 1 2 3 4 5 ○ ○ ○ ○ ○

Energy level 1 2 3 4 5 ○ ○ ○ ○ ○   **Stress level** 1 2 3 4 5 ○ ○ ○ ○ ○

Hours of sleep ☐   **Sleep quality** 1 2 3 4 5 ○ ○ ○ ○ ○

Injuries or illnesses

kJ/Cal intake

Planned kJ/Cal	
Actual kJ/Cal	
Difference [+/-]	

Weight at end of week

BMI at end of week

EXERCISE DIARY

STRENGTH TRAINING		SET 1		SET 2		SET 3		SET4			
Exercise	Focus area	Reps	Weight	Reps	Weight	Reps	Weight	Reps	Weight	Equipment	Ease

CARDIO TRAINING

Exercise	Time	Distance	Intensity	Heart rate	Ease	kJ/Cal burnt

Total kJ/Cal burnt

INCIDENTAL EXERCISE

Day	Activity	Day	Activity

WEEK BEGINNING   /   /

Weight at start of week

BMI at start of week

Planned kJ/Cal this week

Possible diet-busting occasions this week

Planned exercise sessions this week

	Exercise	Completed [Y/N]
Monday		
Tuesday		
Wednesday		
Thursday		
Friday		
Saturday		
Sunday		

FOOD DIARY

MONDAY

	Time		Quantity	Fat	Protein	Carbs	Fibre	kJ/Cal
Breakfast 1 2 3 4 5 ○ ○ ○ ○ ○ HUNGER SCALE								
Mid-morning ○ ○ ○ ○ ○								
Lunch 1 2 3 4 5 ○ ○ ○ ○ ○ HUNGER SCALE								
Mid-afternoon ○ ○ ○ ○ ○								
Dinner 1 2 3 4 5 ○ ○ ○ ○ ○ HUNGER SCALE								
Evening ○ ○ ○ ○ ○								

Coffees/teas   Fluid intake ▽ ▽ ▽ ▽ ▽ ▽ ▽ ▽ ▽ ▽   Daily totals

TUESDAY

	Time		Quantity	Fat	Protein	Carbs	Fibre	kJ/Cal
Breakfast 1 2 3 4 5 ○ ○ ○ ○ ○ HUNGER SCALE								
Mid-morning ○ ○ ○ ○ ○								
Lunch 1 2 3 4 5 ○ ○ ○ ○ ○ HUNGER SCALE								
Mid-afternoon ○ ○ ○ ○ ○								
Dinner 1 2 3 4 5 ○ ○ ○ ○ ○ HUNGER SCALE								
Evening ○ ○ ○ ○ ○								

Coffees/teas   Fluid intake ▽ ▽ ▽ ▽ ▽ ▽ ▽ ▽ ▽ ▽   Daily totals

WEDNESDAY

	Time		Quantity	Fat	Protein	Carbs	Fibre	kJ/Cal
Breakfast 1 2 3 4 5 ○ ○ ○ ○ ○ HUNGER SCALE								
Mid-morning ○ ○ ○ ○ ○								
Lunch 1 2 3 4 5 ○ ○ ○ ○ ○ HUNGER SCALE								
Mid-afternoon ○ ○ ○ ○ ○								
Dinner 1 2 3 4 5 ○ ○ ○ ○ ○ HUNGER SCALE								
Evening ○ ○ ○ ○ ○								

Coffees/teas   Fluid intake ⊔ ⊔ ⊔ ⊔ ⊔ ⊔ ⊔ ⊔ ⊔ ⊔   Daily totals

THURSDAY

	Time		Quantity	Fat	Protein	Carbs	Fibre	kJ/Cal
Breakfast 1 2 3 4 5 ○ ○ ○ ○ ○ HUNGER SCALE								
Mid-morning ○ ○ ○ ○ ○								
Lunch 1 2 3 4 5 ○ ○ ○ ○ ○ HUNGER SCALE								
Mid-afternoon ○ ○ ○ ○ ○								
Dinner 1 2 3 4 5 ○ ○ ○ ○ ○ HUNGER SCALE								
Evening ○ ○ ○ ○ ○								

Coffees/teas   Fluid intake ⊔ ⊔ ⊔ ⊔ ⊔ ⊔ ⊔ ⊔ ⊔ ⊔   Daily totals

FRIDAY

	Time		Quantity	Fat	Protein	Carbs	Fibre	kJ/Cal
Breakfast 1 2 3 4 5 ○ ○ ○ ○ ○ HUNGER SCALE								
Mid-morning ○ ○ ○ ○ ○								
Lunch 1 2 3 4 5 ○ ○ ○ ○ ○ HUNGER SCALE								
Mid-afternoon ○ ○ ○ ○ ○								
Dinner 1 2 3 4 5 ○ ○ ○ ○ ○ HUNGER SCALE								
Evening ○ ○ ○ ○ ○								

Coffees/teas   Fluid intake ⊔ ⊔ ⊔ ⊔ ⊔ ⊔ ⊔ ⊔ ⊔ ⊔   Daily totals

SATURDAY

	Time		Quantity	Fat	Protein	Carbs	Fibre	kJ/Cal
Breakfast 1 2 3 4 5 ○○○○○ HUNGER SCALE								
Mid-morning ○○○○○								
Lunch 1 2 3 4 5 ○○○○○ HUNGER SCALE								
Mid-afternoon ○○○○○								
Dinner 1 2 3 4 5 ○○○○○ HUNGER SCALE								
Evening ○○○○○								

Coffees/teas ☐   Fluid intake ▽▽▽▽▽▽▽▽▽▽   Daily totals

SUNDAY

	Time		Quantity	Fat	Protein	Carbs	Fibre	kJ/Cal
Breakfast 1 2 3 4 5 ○○○○○ HUNGER SCALE								
Mid-morning ○○○○○								
Lunch 1 2 3 4 5 ○○○○○ HUNGER SCALE								
Mid-afternoon ○○○○○								
Dinner 1 2 3 4 5 ○○○○○ HUNGER SCALE								
Evening ○○○○○								

Coffees/teas ☐   Fluid intake ▽▽▽▽▽▽▽▽▽▽   Daily totals

Units of alcohol this week ☐   Total alcohol kJ/Cal ☐

Vitamins and supplements					

	Fat	Protein	Carbs	Fibre	kJ/Cal
WEEKLY TOTALS					

WEEKLY PERSONAL SUMMARY

Mood 1 2 3 4 5 ○○○○○   **Appetite** 1 2 3 4 5 ○○○○○

Energy level 1 2 3 4 5 ○○○○○   **Stress level** 1 2 3 4 5 ○○○○○

Hours of sleep ☐   **Sleep quality** 1 2 3 4 5 ○○○○○

Injuries or illnesses

kJ/Cal intake

Planned kJ/Cal	
Actual kJ/Cal	

Difference [+/-]

Weight at end of week ☐

BMI at end of week ☐

EXERCISE DIARY

STRENGTH TRAINING		SET 1		SET 2		SET 3		SET4			
Exercise	Focus area	Reps	Weight	Reps	Weight	Reps	Weight	Reps	Weight	Equipment	Ease

CARDIO TRAINING

Exercise	Time	Distance	Intensity	Heart rate	Ease	kJ/Cal burnt

Total kJ/Cal burnt

INCIDENTAL EXERCISE

Day	Activity	Day	Activity

WEEK BEGINNING / /

Weight at start of week

BMI at start of week

Planned kJ/Cal this week

Possible diet-busting occasions this week

Planned exercise sessions this week

	Exercise	Completed [Y/N]
Monday		
Tuesday		
Wednesday		
Thursday		
Friday		
Saturday		
Sunday		

FOOD DIARY

MONDAY

	Time		Quantity	Fat	Protein	Carbs	Fibre	kJ/Cal
Breakfast 1 2 3 4 5 ○ ○ ○ ○ ○ HUNGER SCALE								
Mid-morning ○ ○ ○ ○ ○								
Lunch 1 2 3 4 5 ○ ○ ○ ○ ○ HUNGER SCALE								
Mid-afternoon ○ ○ ○ ○ ○								
Dinner 1 2 3 4 5 ○ ○ ○ ○ ○ HUNGER SCALE								
Evening ○ ○ ○ ○ ○								

Coffees/teas   Fluid intake ▽▽▽▽▽▽▽▽▽▽ Daily totals

TUESDAY

	Time		Quantity	Fat	Protein	Carbs	Fibre	kJ/Cal
Breakfast 1 2 3 4 5 ○ ○ ○ ○ ○ HUNGER SCALE								
Mid-morning ○ ○ ○ ○ ○								
Lunch 1 2 3 4 5 ○ ○ ○ ○ ○ HUNGER SCALE								
Mid-afternoon ○ ○ ○ ○ ○								
Dinner 1 2 3 4 5 ○ ○ ○ ○ ○ HUNGER SCALE								
Evening ○ ○ ○ ○ ○								

Coffees/teas   Fluid intake ▽▽▽▽▽▽▽▽▽▽ Daily totals

WEDNESDAY

	Time		Quantity	Fat	Protein	Carbs	Fibre	kJ/Cal
Breakfast 1 2 3 4 5 ○ ○ ○ ○ ○ HUNGER SCALE								
Mid-morning ○ ○ ○ ○ ○								
Lunch 1 2 3 4 5 ○ ○ ○ ○ ○ HUNGER SCALE								
Mid-afternoon ○ ○ ○ ○ ○								
Dinner 1 2 3 4 5 ○ ○ ○ ○ ○ HUNGER SCALE								
Evening ○ ○ ○ ○ ○								

Coffees/teas ___ Fluid intake ☐☐☐☐☐☐☐☐☐☐ Daily totals

THURSDAY

	Time		Quantity	Fat	Protein	Carbs	Fibre	kJ/Cal
Breakfast 1 2 3 4 5 ○ ○ ○ ○ ○ HUNGER SCALE								
Mid-morning ○ ○ ○ ○ ○								
Lunch 1 2 3 4 5 ○ ○ ○ ○ ○ HUNGER SCALE								
Mid-afternoon ○ ○ ○ ○ ○								
Dinner 1 2 3 4 5 ○ ○ ○ ○ ○ HUNGER SCALE								
Evening ○ ○ ○ ○ ○								

Coffees/teas ___ Fluid intake ☐☐☐☐☐☐☐☐☐☐ Daily totals

FRIDAY

	Time		Quantity	Fat	Protein	Carbs	Fibre	kJ/Cal
Breakfast 1 2 3 4 5 ○ ○ ○ ○ ○ HUNGER SCALE								
Mid-morning ○ ○ ○ ○ ○								
Lunch 1 2 3 4 5 ○ ○ ○ ○ ○ HUNGER SCALE								
Mid-afternoon ○ ○ ○ ○ ○								
Dinner 1 2 3 4 5 ○ ○ ○ ○ ○ HUNGER SCALE								
Evening ○ ○ ○ ○ ○								

Coffees/teas ___ Fluid intake ☐☐☐☐☐☐☐☐☐☐ Daily totals

SATURDAY

	Time				Quantity	Fat	Protein	Carbs	Fibre	kJ/Cal
Breakfast 1 2 3 4 5 ○ ○ ○ ○ ○ HUNGER SCALE										
Mid-morning ○ ○ ○ ○ ○										
Lunch 1 2 3 4 5 ○ ○ ○ ○ ○ HUNGER SCALE										
Mid-afternoon ○ ○ ○ ○ ○										
Dinner 1 2 3 4 5 ○ ○ ○ ○ ○ HUNGER SCALE										
Evening ○ ○ ○ ○ ○										

Coffees/teas ☐   Fluid intake ⌒⌒⌒⌒⌒⌒⌒⌒⌒⌒   Daily totals

SUNDAY

	Time				Quantity	Fat	Protein	Carbs	Fibre	kJ/Cal
Breakfast 1 2 3 4 5 ○ ○ ○ ○ ○ HUNGER SCALE										
Mid-morning ○ ○ ○ ○ ○										
Lunch 1 2 3 4 5 ○ ○ ○ ○ ○ HUNGER SCALE										
Mid-afternoon ○ ○ ○ ○ ○										
Dinner 1 2 3 4 5 ○ ○ ○ ○ ○ HUNGER SCALE										
Evening ○ ○ ○ ○ ○										

Coffees/teas ☐   Fluid intake ⌒⌒⌒⌒⌒⌒⌒⌒⌒⌒   Daily totals

Units of alcohol this week ☐   Total alcohol kJ/Cal ☐

Vitamins and supplements

WEEKLY TOTALS	Fat	Protein	Carbs	Fibre	kJ/Cal

WEEKLY PERSONAL SUMMARY

Mood 1 2 3 4 5 ○ ○ ○ ○ ○   Appetite 1 2 3 4 5 ○ ○ ○ ○ ○

Energy level 1 2 3 4 5 ○ ○ ○ ○ ○   Stress level 1 2 3 4 5 ○ ○ ○ ○ ○

Hours of sleep ☐   Sleep quality 1 2 3 4 5 ○ ○ ○ ○ ○

kJ/Cal intake

Planned kJ/Cal	
Actual kJ/Cal	

Difference [+/-]

Weight at end of week ☐

BMI at end of week ☐

Injuries or illnesses

EXERCISE DIARY

STRENGTH TRAINING

Exercise	Focus area	SET 1		SET 2		SET 3		SET4		Equipment	Ease
		Reps	Weight	Reps	Weight	Reps	Weight	Reps	Weight		

CARDIO TRAINING

Exercise	Time	Distance	Intensity	Heart rate	Ease	kJ/Cal burnt

Total kJ/Cal burnt

INCIDENTAL EXERCISE

Day	Activity	Day	Activity

WEEK BEGINNING   /   /

Weight at start of week

BMI at start of week

Planned kJ/Cal this week

Possible diet-busting occasions this week

Planned exercise sessions this week

	Exercise	Completed [Y/N]
Monday		
Tuesday		
Wednesday		
Thursday		
Friday		
Saturday		
Sunday		

FOOD DIARY

MONDAY

	Time		Quantity	Fat	Protein	Carbs	Fibre	kJ/Cal
Breakfast 1 2 3 4 5 ○ ○ ○ ○ ○ HUNGER SCALE								
Mid-morning ○ ○ ○ ○ ○								
Lunch 1 2 3 4 5 ○ ○ ○ ○ ○ HUNGER SCALE								
Mid-afternoon ○ ○ ○ ○ ○								
Dinner 1 2 3 4 5 ○ ○ ○ ○ ○ HUNGER SCALE								
Evening ○ ○ ○ ○ ○								

Coffees/teas   Fluid intake ⊔⊔⊔⊔⊔⊔⊔⊔⊔⊔   Daily totals

TUESDAY

			Quantity	Fat	Protein	Carbs	Fibre	kJ/Cal
Breakfast 1 2 3 4 5 ○ ○ ○ ○ ○ HUNGER SCALE								
Mid-morning ○ ○ ○ ○ ○								
Lunch 1 2 3 4 5 ○ ○ ○ ○ ○ HUNGER SCALE								
Mid-afternoon ○ ○ ○ ○ ○								
Dinner 1 2 3 4 5 ○ ○ ○ ○ ○ HUNGER SCALE								
Evening ○ ○ ○ ○ ○								

Coffees/teas   Fluid intake ⊔⊔⊔⊔⊔⊔⊔⊔⊔⊔   Daily totals

WEDNESDAY

	Time		Quantity	Fat	Protein	Carbs	Fibre	kJ/Cal
Breakfast 1 2 3 4 5 ○ ○ ○ ○ ○ HUNGER SCALE								
Mid-morning ○ ○ ○ ○ ○								
Lunch 1 2 3 4 5 ○ ○ ○ ○ ○ HUNGER SCALE								
Mid-afternoon ○ ○ ○ ○ ○								
Dinner 1 2 3 4 5 ○ ○ ○ ○ ○ HUNGER SCALE								
Evening ○ ○ ○ ○ ○								

Coffees/teas　　　Fluid intake ▢▢▢▢▢▢▢▢▢▢　Daily totals

THURSDAY

	Time		Quantity	Fat	Protein	Carbs	Fibre	kJ/Cal
Breakfast 1 2 3 4 5 ○ ○ ○ ○ ○ HUNGER SCALE								
Mid-morning ○ ○ ○ ○ ○								
Lunch 1 2 3 4 5 ○ ○ ○ ○ ○ HUNGER SCALE								
Mid-afternoon ○ ○ ○ ○ ○								
Dinner 1 2 3 4 5 ○ ○ ○ ○ ○ HUNGER SCALE								
Evening ○ ○ ○ ○ ○								

Coffees/teas　　　Fluid intake ▢▢▢▢▢▢▢▢▢▢　Daily totals

FRIDAY

	Time		Quantity	Fat	Protein	Carbs	Fibre	kJ/Cal
Breakfast 1 2 3 4 5 ○ ○ ○ ○ ○ HUNGER SCALE								
Mid-morning ○ ○ ○ ○ ○								
Lunch 1 2 3 4 5 ○ ○ ○ ○ ○ HUNGER SCALE								
Mid-afternoon ○ ○ ○ ○ ○								
Dinner 1 2 3 4 5 ○ ○ ○ ○ ○ HUNGER SCALE								
Evening ○ ○ ○ ○ ○								

Coffees/teas　　　Fluid intake ▢▢▢▢▢▢▢▢▢▢　Daily totals

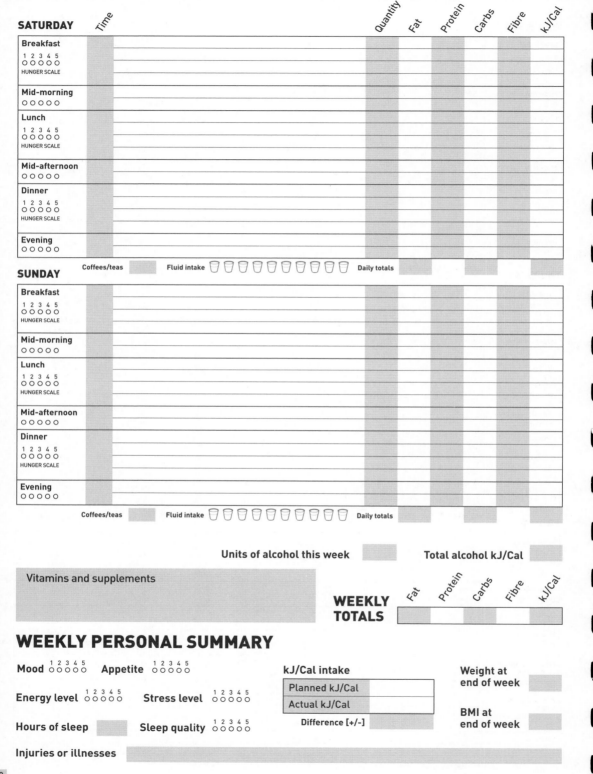

SATURDAY

	Time		Quantity	Fat	Protein	Carbs	Fibre	kJ/Cal
Breakfast 1 2 3 4 5 ○ ○ ○ ○ ○ HUNGER SCALE								
Mid-morning ○ ○ ○ ○ ○								
Lunch 1 2 3 4 5 ○ ○ ○ ○ ○ HUNGER SCALE								
Mid-afternoon ○ ○ ○ ○ ○								
Dinner 1 2 3 4 5 ○ ○ ○ ○ ○ HUNGER SCALE								
Evening ○ ○ ○ ○ ○								

Coffees/teas   Fluid intake ⌄⌄⌄⌄⌄⌄⌄⌄⌄⌄   Daily totals

SUNDAY

	Time		Quantity	Fat	Protein	Carbs	Fibre	kJ/Cal
Breakfast 1 2 3 4 5 ○ ○ ○ ○ ○ HUNGER SCALE								
Mid-morning ○ ○ ○ ○ ○								
Lunch 1 2 3 4 5 ○ ○ ○ ○ ○ HUNGER SCALE								
Mid-afternoon ○ ○ ○ ○ ○								
Dinner 1 2 3 4 5 ○ ○ ○ ○ ○ HUNGER SCALE								
Evening ○ ○ ○ ○ ○								

Coffees/teas   Fluid intake ⌄⌄⌄⌄⌄⌄⌄⌄⌄⌄   Daily totals

Units of alcohol this week   Total alcohol kJ/Cal

Vitamins and supplements

WEEKLY TOTALS	Fat	Protein	Carbs	Fibre	kJ/Cal

WEEKLY PERSONAL SUMMARY

Mood 1 2 3 4 5 ○ ○ ○ ○ ○   **Appetite** 1 2 3 4 5 ○ ○ ○ ○ ○

Energy level 1 2 3 4 5 ○ ○ ○ ○ ○   **Stress level** 1 2 3 4 5 ○ ○ ○ ○ ○

Hours of sleep   **Sleep quality** 1 2 3 4 5 ○ ○ ○ ○ ○

kJ/Cal intake	
Planned kJ/Cal	
Actual kJ/Cal	
Difference [+/-]	

Weight at end of week

BMI at end of week

Injuries or illnesses

EXERCISE DIARY

STRENGTH TRAINING		SET 1		SET 2		SET 3		SET4			
Exercise	Focus area	Reps	Weight	Reps	Weight	Reps	Weight	Reps	Weight	Equipment	Ease

CARDIO TRAINING

Exercise	Time	Distance	Intensity	Heart rate	Ease	kJ/Cal burnt

Total kJ/Cal burnt

INCIDENTAL EXERCISE

Day	Activity	Day	Activity

WEEK BEGINNING ___ / ___ / ___

Weight at start of week ___

BMI at start of week ___

Planned kJ/Cal this week ___

Possible diet-busting occasions this week

___

Planned exercise sessions this week

	Exercise	Completed [Y/N]
Monday		
Tuesday		
Wednesday		
Thursday		
Friday		
Saturday		
Sunday		

FOOD DIARY

MONDAY

Time		Quantity	Fat	Protein	Carbs	Fibre	kJ/Cal
Breakfast 1 2 3 4 5 ○○○○○ HUNGER SCALE							
Mid-morning ○○○○○							
Lunch 1 2 3 4 5 ○○○○○ HUNGER SCALE							
Mid-afternoon ○○○○○							
Dinner 1 2 3 4 5 ○○○○○ HUNGER SCALE							
Evening ○○○○○							

Coffees/teas ___ Fluid intake ☐☐☐☐☐☐☐☐☐☐ Daily totals

TUESDAY

Time		Quantity	Fat	Protein	Carbs	Fibre	kJ/Cal
Breakfast 1 2 3 4 5 ○○○○○ HUNGER SCALE							
Mid-morning ○○○○○							
Lunch 1 2 3 4 5 ○○○○○ HUNGER SCALE							
Mid-afternoon ○○○○○							
Dinner 1 2 3 4 5 ○○○○○ HUNGER SCALE							
Evening ○○○○○							

Coffees/teas ___ Fluid intake ☐☐☐☐☐☐☐☐☐☐ Daily totals

WEDNESDAY

	Time		Quantity	Fat	Protein	Carbs	Fibre	kJ/Cal
Breakfast 1 2 3 4 5 ○ ○ ○ ○ ○ HUNGER SCALE								
Mid-morning ○ ○ ○ ○ ○								
Lunch 1 2 3 4 5 ○ ○ ○ ○ ○ HUNGER SCALE								
Mid-afternoon ○ ○ ○ ○ ○								
Dinner 1 2 3 4 5 ○ ○ ○ ○ ○ HUNGER SCALE								
Evening ○ ○ ○ ○ ○								

Coffees/teas   Fluid intake ☐☐☐☐☐☐☐☐☐☐   Daily totals

THURSDAY

	Time		Quantity	Fat	Protein	Carbs	Fibre	kJ/Cal
Breakfast 1 2 3 4 5 ○ ○ ○ ○ ○ HUNGER SCALE								
Mid-morning ○ ○ ○ ○ ○								
Lunch 1 2 3 4 5 ○ ○ ○ ○ ○ HUNGER SCALE								
Mid-afternoon ○ ○ ○ ○ ○								
Dinner 1 2 3 4 5 ○ ○ ○ ○ ○ HUNGER SCALE								
Evening ○ ○ ○ ○ ○								

Coffees/teas   Fluid intake ☐☐☐☐☐☐☐☐☐☐   Daily totals

FRIDAY

	Time		Quantity	Fat	Protein	Carbs	Fibre	kJ/Cal
Breakfast 1 2 3 4 5 ○ ○ ○ ○ ○ HUNGER SCALE								
Mid-morning ○ ○ ○ ○ ○								
Lunch 1 2 3 4 5 ○ ○ ○ ○ ○ HUNGER SCALE								
Mid-afternoon ○ ○ ○ ○ ○								
Dinner 1 2 3 4 5 ○ ○ ○ ○ ○ HUNGER SCALE								
Evening ○ ○ ○ ○ ○								

Coffees/teas   Fluid intake ☐☐☐☐☐☐☐☐☐☐   Daily totals

SATURDAY

	Time		Quantity	Fat	Protein	Carbs	Fibre	kJ/Cal
Breakfast 1 2 3 4 5 ○○○○○ HUNGER SCALE								
Mid-morning ○○○○○								
Lunch 1 2 3 4 5 ○○○○○ HUNGER SCALE								
Mid-afternoon ○○○○○								
Dinner 1 2 3 4 5 ○○○○○ HUNGER SCALE								
Evening ○○○○○								

Coffees/teas   Fluid intake ▽▽▽▽▽▽▽▽▽▽   Daily totals

SUNDAY

	Time		Quantity	Fat	Protein	Carbs	Fibre	kJ/Cal
Breakfast 1 2 3 4 5 ○○○○○ HUNGER SCALE								
Mid-morning ○○○○○								
Lunch 1 2 3 4 5 ○○○○○ HUNGER SCALE								
Mid-afternoon ○○○○○								
Dinner 1 2 3 4 5 ○○○○○ HUNGER SCALE								
Evening ○○○○○								

Coffees/teas   Fluid intake ▽▽▽▽▽▽▽▽▽▽   Daily totals

Units of alcohol this week   **Total alcohol kJ/Cal**

Vitamins and supplements

WEEKLY TOTALS	Fat	Protein	Carbs	Fibre	kJ/Cal

WEEKLY PERSONAL SUMMARY

Mood 1 2 3 4 5 ○○○○○   **Appetite** 1 2 3 4 5 ○○○○○

Energy level 1 2 3 4 5 ○○○○○   **Stress level** 1 2 3 4 5 ○○○○○

Hours of sleep [ ]   **Sleep quality** 1 2 3 4 5 ○○○○○

kJ/Cal intake

Planned kJ/Cal	
Actual kJ/Cal	

Difference [+/-]

Weight at end of week

BMI at end of week

Injuries or illnesses

EXERCISE DIARY

STRENGTH TRAINING		SET 1		SET 2		SET 3		SET4			
Exercise	Focus area	Reps	Weight	Reps	Weight	Reps	Weight	Reps	Weight	Equipment	Ease

CARDIO TRAINING

Exercise	Time	Distance	Intensity	Heart rate	Ease	kJ/Cal burnt

Total kJ/Cal burnt

INCIDENTAL EXERCISE

Day	Activity	Day	Activity

WEEK BEGINNING   /   /

Weight at start of week

BMI at start of week

Planned kJ/Cal this week

Possible diet-busting occasions this week

Planned exercise sessions this week

	Exercise	Completed [Y/N]
Monday		
Tuesday		
Wednesday		
Thursday		
Friday		
Saturday		
Sunday		

FOOD DIARY

MONDAY

	Time		Quantity	Fat	Protein	Carbs	Fibre	kJ/Cal
Breakfast 1 2 3 4 5 ○ ○ ○ ○ ○ HUNGER SCALE								
Mid-morning ○ ○ ○ ○ ○								
Lunch 1 2 3 4 5 ○ ○ ○ ○ ○ HUNGER SCALE								
Mid-afternoon ○ ○ ○ ○ ○								
Dinner 1 2 3 4 5 ○ ○ ○ ○ ○ HUNGER SCALE								
Evening ○ ○ ○ ○ ○								

Coffees/teas   Fluid intake ☐☐☐☐☐☐☐☐☐☐ Daily totals

TUESDAY

	Time		Quantity	Fat	Protein	Carbs	Fibre	kJ/Cal
Breakfast 1 2 3 4 5 ○ ○ ○ ○ ○ HUNGER SCALE								
Mid-morning ○ ○ ○ ○ ○								
Lunch 1 2 3 4 5 ○ ○ ○ ○ ○ HUNGER SCALE								
Mid-afternoon ○ ○ ○ ○ ○								
Dinner 1 2 3 4 5 ○ ○ ○ ○ ○ HUNGER SCALE								
Evening ○ ○ ○ ○ ○								

Coffees/teas   Fluid intake ☐☐☐☐☐☐☐☐☐☐ Daily totals

WEDNESDAY

	Time		Quantity	Fat	Protein	Carbs	Fibre	kJ/Cal
Breakfast 1 2 3 4 5 ○○○○○ HUNGER SCALE								
Mid-morning ○○○○○								
Lunch 1 2 3 4 5 ○○○○○ HUNGER SCALE								
Mid-afternoon ○○○○○								
Dinner 1 2 3 4 5 ○○○○○ HUNGER SCALE								
Evening ○○○○○								

Coffees/teas ☐ Fluid intake ⊔⊔⊔⊔⊔⊔⊔⊔⊔⊔ Daily totals

THURSDAY

	Time		Quantity	Fat	Protein	Carbs	Fibre	kJ/Cal
Breakfast 1 2 3 4 5 ○○○○○ HUNGER SCALE								
Mid-morning ○○○○○								
Lunch 1 2 3 4 5 ○○○○○ HUNGER SCALE								
Mid-afternoon ○○○○○								
Dinner 1 2 3 4 5 ○○○○○ HUNGER SCALE								
Evening ○○○○○								

Coffees/teas ☐ Fluid intake ⊔⊔⊔⊔⊔⊔⊔⊔⊔⊔ Daily totals

FRIDAY

	Time		Quantity	Fat	Protein	Carbs	Fibre	kJ/Cal
Breakfast 1 2 3 4 5 ○○○○○ HUNGER SCALE								
Mid-morning ○○○○○								
Lunch 1 2 3 4 5 ○○○○○ HUNGER SCALE								
Mid-afternoon ○○○○○								
Dinner 1 2 3 4 5 ○○○○○ HUNGER SCALE								
Evening ○○○○○								

Coffees/teas ☐ Fluid intake ⊔⊔⊔⊔⊔⊔⊔⊔⊔⊔ Daily totals

SATURDAY

	Time		Quantity	Fat	Protein	Carbs	Fibre	kJ/Cal
Breakfast 1 2 3 4 5 ○○○○○ HUNGER SCALE								
Mid-morning ○○○○○								
Lunch 1 2 3 4 5 ○○○○○ HUNGER SCALE								
Mid-afternoon ○○○○○								
Dinner 1 2 3 4 5 ○○○○○ HUNGER SCALE								
Evening ○○○○○								

Coffees/teas [ ]   Fluid intake ⛾⛾⛾⛾⛾⛾⛾⛾⛾⛾   Daily totals

SUNDAY

	Time		Quantity	Fat	Protein	Carbs	Fibre	kJ/Cal
Breakfast 1 2 3 4 5 ○○○○○ HUNGER SCALE								
Mid-morning ○○○○○								
Lunch 1 2 3 4 5 ○○○○○ HUNGER SCALE								
Mid-afternoon ○○○○○								
Dinner 1 2 3 4 5 ○○○○○ HUNGER SCALE								
Evening ○○○○○								

Coffees/teas [ ]   Fluid intake ⛾⛾⛾⛾⛾⛾⛾⛾⛾⛾   Daily totals

Units of alcohol this week [ ]   Total alcohol kJ/Cal [ ]

Vitamins and supplements

WEEKLY TOTALS	Fat	Protein	Carbs	Fibre	kJ/Cal

WEEKLY PERSONAL SUMMARY

Mood 1 2 3 4 5 ○○○○○   **Appetite** 1 2 3 4 5 ○○○○○

Energy level 1 2 3 4 5 ○○○○○   **Stress level** 1 2 3 4 5 ○○○○○

Hours of sleep [ ]   **Sleep quality** 1 2 3 4 5 ○○○○○

Injuries or illnesses [ ]

kJ/Cal intake

Planned kJ/Cal	
Actual kJ/Cal	
Difference [+/-]	

Weight at end of week [ ]

BMI at end of week [ ]

EXERCISE DIARY

STRENGTH TRAINING		SET 1		SET 2		SET 3		SET4			
Exercise	Focus area	Reps	Weight	Reps	Weight	Reps	Weight	Reps	Weight	Equipment	Ease

CARDIO TRAINING

Exercise	Time	Distance	Intensity	Heart rate	Ease	kJ/Cal burnt

Total kJ/Cal burnt

INCIDENTAL EXERCISE

Day	Activity	Day	Activity

WEEK BEGINNING / /

Weight at start of week

BMI at start of week

Planned kJ/Cal this week

Possible diet-busting occasions this week

Planned exercise sessions this week

	Exercise	Completed [Y/N]
Monday		
Tuesday		
Wednesday		
Thursday		
Friday		
Saturday		
Sunday		

FOOD DIARY

MONDAY

	Time		Quantity	Fat	Protein	Carbs	Fibre	kJ/Cal
Breakfast 1 2 3 4 5 ○ ○ ○ ○ ○ HUNGER SCALE								
Mid-morning ○ ○ ○ ○ ○								
Lunch 1 2 3 4 5 ○ ○ ○ ○ ○ HUNGER SCALE								
Mid-afternoon ○ ○ ○ ○ ○								
Dinner 1 2 3 4 5 ○ ○ ○ ○ ○ HUNGER SCALE								
Evening ○ ○ ○ ○ ○								

Coffees/teas ___ Fluid intake ▽▽▽▽▽▽▽▽▽▽ Daily totals

TUESDAY

	Time		Quantity	Fat	Protein	Carbs	Fibre	kJ/Cal
Breakfast 1 2 3 4 5 ○ ○ ○ ○ ○ HUNGER SCALE								
Mid-morning ○ ○ ○ ○ ○								
Lunch 1 2 3 4 5 ○ ○ ○ ○ ○ HUNGER SCALE								
Mid-afternoon ○ ○ ○ ○ ○								
Dinner 1 2 3 4 5 ○ ○ ○ ○ ○ HUNGER SCALE								
Evening ○ ○ ○ ○ ○								

Coffees/teas ___ Fluid intake ▽▽▽▽▽▽▽▽▽▽ Daily totals

WEDNESDAY

	Time		Quantity	Fat	Protein	Carbs	Fibre	kJ/Cal
Breakfast 1 2 3 4 5 ○ ○ ○ ○ ○ HUNGER SCALE								
Mid-morning ○ ○ ○ ○ ○								
Lunch 1 2 3 4 5 ○ ○ ○ ○ ○ HUNGER SCALE								
Mid-afternoon ○ ○ ○ ○ ○								
Dinner 1 2 3 4 5 ○ ○ ○ ○ ○ HUNGER SCALE								
Evening ○ ○ ○ ○ ○								

Coffees/teas ☐   Fluid intake ▽▽▽▽▽▽▽▽▽▽   Daily totals

THURSDAY

	Time		Quantity	Fat	Protein	Carbs	Fibre	kJ/Cal
Breakfast 1 2 3 4 5 ○ ○ ○ ○ ○ HUNGER SCALE								
Mid-morning ○ ○ ○ ○ ○								
Lunch 1 2 3 4 5 ○ ○ ○ ○ ○ HUNGER SCALE								
Mid-afternoon ○ ○ ○ ○ ○								
Dinner 1 2 3 4 5 ○ ○ ○ ○ ○ HUNGER SCALE								
Evening ○ ○ ○ ○ ○								

Coffees/teas ☐   Fluid intake ▽▽▽▽▽▽▽▽▽▽   Daily totals

FRIDAY

	Time		Quantity	Fat	Protein	Carbs	Fibre	kJ/Cal
Breakfast 1 2 3 4 5 ○ ○ ○ ○ ○ HUNGER SCALE								
Mid-morning ○ ○ ○ ○ ○								
Lunch 1 2 3 4 5 ○ ○ ○ ○ ○ HUNGER SCALE								
Mid-afternoon ○ ○ ○ ○ ○								
Dinner 1 2 3 4 5 ○ ○ ○ ○ ○ HUNGER SCALE								
Evening ○ ○ ○ ○ ○								

Coffees/teas ☐   Fluid intake ▽▽▽▽▽▽▽▽▽▽   Daily totals

SATURDAY

	Time		Quantity	Fat	Protein	Carbs	Fibre	kJ/Cal
Breakfast 1 2 3 4 5 ○○○○○ HUNGER SCALE								
Mid-morning ○○○○○								
Lunch 1 2 3 4 5 ○○○○○ HUNGER SCALE								
Mid-afternoon ○○○○○								
Dinner 1 2 3 4 5 ○○○○○ HUNGER SCALE								
Evening ○○○○○								

Coffees/teas ▢   Fluid intake ▢▢▢▢▢▢▢▢▢▢   Daily totals

SUNDAY

	Time		Quantity	Fat	Protein	Carbs	Fibre	kJ/Cal
Breakfast 1 2 3 4 5 ○○○○○ HUNGER SCALE								
Mid-morning ○○○○○								
Lunch 1 2 3 4 5 ○○○○○ HUNGER SCALE								
Mid-afternoon ○○○○○								
Dinner 1 2 3 4 5 ○○○○○ HUNGER SCALE								
Evening ○○○○○								

Coffees/teas ▢   Fluid intake ▢▢▢▢▢▢▢▢▢▢   Daily totals

Units of alcohol this week ▢   Total alcohol kJ/Cal ▢

Vitamins and supplements

		Fat	Protein	Carbs	Fibre	kJ/Cal
WEEKLY TOTALS						

WEEKLY PERSONAL SUMMARY

Mood 1 2 3 4 5 ○○○○○   **Appetite** 1 2 3 4 5 ○○○○○

Energy level 1 2 3 4 5 ○○○○○   **Stress level** 1 2 3 4 5 ○○○○○

Hours of sleep ▢   **Sleep quality** 1 2 3 4 5 ○○○○○

Injuries or illnesses

kJ/Cal intake

Planned kJ/Cal	
Actual kJ/Cal	

Difference [+/-]

Weight at end of week

BMI at end of week

EXERCISE DIARY

STRENGTH TRAINING		SET 1		SET 2		SET 3		SET4			
Exercise	Focus area	Reps	Weight	Reps	Weight	Reps	Weight	Reps	Weight	Equipment	Ease

CARDIO TRAINING

Exercise	Time	Distance	Intensity	Heart rate	Ease	kJ/Cal burnt

Total kJ/Cal burnt

INCIDENTAL EXERCISE

Day	Activity	Day	Activity

WEEK BEGINNING ⬚ / ⬚ / ⬚

Weight at start of week ⬚

BMI at start of week ⬚

Planned kJ/Cal this week ⬚

Possible diet-busting occasions this week

⬚

Planned exercise sessions this week

	Exercise	Completed [Y/N]
Monday		
Tuesday		
Wednesday		
Thursday		
Friday		
Saturday		
Sunday		

FOOD DIARY

MONDAY

	Time		Quantity	Fat	Protein	Carbs	Fibre	kJ/Cal
Breakfast 1 2 3 4 5 ○○○○○ HUNGER SCALE								
Mid-morning ○○○○○								
Lunch 1 2 3 4 5 ○○○○○ HUNGER SCALE								
Mid-afternoon ○○○○○								
Dinner 1 2 3 4 5 ○○○○○ HUNGER SCALE								
Evening ○○○○○								

Coffees/teas ⬚   Fluid intake ▽▽▽▽▽▽▽▽▽▽   Daily totals

TUESDAY

	Time		Quantity	Fat	Protein	Carbs	Fibre	kJ/Cal
Breakfast 1 2 3 4 5 ○○○○○ HUNGER SCALE								
Mid-morning ○○○○○								
Lunch 1 2 3 4 5 ○○○○○ HUNGER SCALE								
Mid-afternoon ○○○○○								
Dinner 1 2 3 4 5 ○○○○○ HUNGER SCALE								
Evening ○○○○○								

Coffees/teas ⬚   Fluid intake ▽▽▽▽▽▽▽▽▽▽   Daily totals

WEDNESDAY

	Time		Quantity	Fat	Protein	Carbs	Fibre	kJ/Cal
Breakfast								
1 2 3 4 5 ○○○○○ HUNGER SCALE								
Mid-morning ○○○○○								
Lunch								
1 2 3 4 5 ○○○○○ HUNGER SCALE								
Mid-afternoon ○○○○○								
Dinner								
1 2 3 4 5 ○○○○○ HUNGER SCALE								
Evening ○○○○○								

Coffees/teas   Fluid intake ▭▭▭▭▭▭▭▭▭▭   Daily totals

THURSDAY

	Time		Quantity	Fat	Protein	Carbs	Fibre	kJ/Cal
Breakfast								
1 2 3 4 5 ○○○○○ HUNGER SCALE								
Mid-morning ○○○○○								
Lunch								
1 2 3 4 5 ○○○○○ HUNGER SCALE								
Mid-afternoon ○○○○○								
Dinner								
1 2 3 4 5 ○○○○○ HUNGER SCALE								
Evening ○○○○○								

Coffees/teas   Fluid intake ▭▭▭▭▭▭▭▭▭▭   Daily totals

FRIDAY

	Time		Quantity	Fat	Protein	Carbs	Fibre	kJ/Cal
Breakfast								
1 2 3 4 5 ○○○○○ HUNGER SCALE								
Mid-morning ○○○○○								
Lunch								
1 2 3 4 5 ○○○○○ HUNGER SCALE								
Mid-afternoon ○○○○○								
Dinner								
1 2 3 4 5 ○○○○○ HUNGER SCALE								
Evening ○○○○○								

Coffees/teas   Fluid intake ▭▭▭▭▭▭▭▭▭▭   Daily totals

SATURDAY

	Time				Quantity	Fat	Protein	Carbs	Fibre	kJ/Cal
Breakfast 1 2 3 4 5 ○○○○○ HUNGER SCALE										
Mid-morning ○○○○○										
Lunch 1 2 3 4 5 ○○○○○ HUNGER SCALE										
Mid-afternoon ○○○○○										
Dinner 1 2 3 4 5 ○○○○○ HUNGER SCALE										
Evening ○○○○○										

Coffees/teas   Fluid intake ⊔⊔⊔⊔⊔⊔⊔⊔⊔⊔   Daily totals

SUNDAY

	Time				Quantity	Fat	Protein	Carbs	Fibre	kJ/Cal
Breakfast 1 2 3 4 5 ○○○○○ HUNGER SCALE										
Mid-morning ○○○○○										
Lunch 1 2 3 4 5 ○○○○○ HUNGER SCALE										
Mid-afternoon ○○○○○										
Dinner 1 2 3 4 5 ○○○○○ HUNGER SCALE										
Evening ○○○○○										

Coffees/teas   Fluid intake ⊔⊔⊔⊔⊔⊔⊔⊔⊔⊔   Daily totals

Units of alcohol this week   **Total alcohol kJ/Cal**

Vitamins and supplements

	Fat	Protein	Carbs	Fibre	kJ/Cal
WEEKLY TOTALS					

WEEKLY PERSONAL SUMMARY

Mood 1 2 3 4 5 ○○○○○   **Appetite** 1 2 3 4 5 ○○○○○

Energy level 1 2 3 4 5 ○○○○○   **Stress level** 1 2 3 4 5 ○○○○○

Hours of sleep   **Sleep quality** 1 2 3 4 5 ○○○○○

Injuries or illnesses

kJ/Cal intake	
Planned kJ/Cal	
Actual kJ/Cal	
Difference [+/-]	

Weight at end of week

BMI at end of week

EXERCISE DIARY

STRENGTH TRAINING		SET 1		SET 2		SET 3		SET4			
Exercise	Focus area	Reps	Weight	Reps	Weight	Reps	Weight	Reps	Weight	Equipment	Ease

CARDIO TRAINING

Exercise	Time	Distance	Intensity	Heart rate	Ease	kJ/Cal burnt

Total kJ/Cal burnt

INCIDENTAL EXERCISE

Day	Activity	Day	Activity

WEEK BEGINNING ___ / ___ / ___

Weight at start of week

BMI at start of week

Planned kJ/Cal this week

Possible diet-busting occasions this week

Planned exercise sessions this week

	Exercise	Completed [Y/N]
Monday		
Tuesday		
Wednesday		
Thursday		
Friday		
Saturday		
Sunday		

FOOD DIARY

MONDAY

Time		Quantity	Fat	Protein	Carbs	Fibre	kJ/Cal
Breakfast 1 2 3 4 5 ○○○○○ HUNGER SCALE							
Mid-morning ○○○○○							
Lunch 1 2 3 4 5 ○○○○○ HUNGER SCALE							
Mid-afternoon ○○○○○							
Dinner 1 2 3 4 5 ○○○○○ HUNGER SCALE							
Evening ○○○○○							

Coffees/teas ___ Fluid intake ▽▽▽▽▽▽▽▽▽▽ Daily totals

TUESDAY

Time		Quantity	Fat	Protein	Carbs	Fibre	kJ/Cal
Breakfast 1 2 3 4 5 ○○○○○ HUNGER SCALE							
Mid-morning ○○○○○							
Lunch 1 2 3 4 5 ○○○○○ HUNGER SCALE							
Mid-afternoon ○○○○○							
Dinner 1 2 3 4 5 ○○○○○ HUNGER SCALE							
Evening ○○○○○							

Coffees/teas ___ Fluid intake ▽▽▽▽▽▽▽▽▽▽ Daily totals

WEDNESDAY

	Time		Quantity	Fat	Protein	Carbs	Fibre	kJ/Cal
Breakfast 1 2 3 4 5 ○ ○ ○ ○ ○ HUNGER SCALE								
Mid-morning ○ ○ ○ ○ ○								
Lunch 1 2 3 4 5 ○ ○ ○ ○ ○ HUNGER SCALE								
Mid-afternoon ○ ○ ○ ○ ○								
Dinner 1 2 3 4 5 ○ ○ ○ ○ ○ HUNGER SCALE								
Evening ○ ○ ○ ○ ○								

Coffees/teas   Fluid intake ⛆⛆⛆⛆⛆⛆⛆⛆⛆⛆   Daily totals

THURSDAY

	Time		Quantity	Fat	Protein	Carbs	Fibre	kJ/Cal
Breakfast 1 2 3 4 5 ○ ○ ○ ○ ○ HUNGER SCALE								
Mid-morning ○ ○ ○ ○ ○								
Lunch 1 2 3 4 5 ○ ○ ○ ○ ○ HUNGER SCALE								
Mid-afternoon ○ ○ ○ ○ ○								
Dinner 1 2 3 4 5 ○ ○ ○ ○ ○ HUNGER SCALE								
Evening ○ ○ ○ ○ ○								

Coffees/teas   Fluid intake ⛆⛆⛆⛆⛆⛆⛆⛆⛆⛆   Daily totals

FRIDAY

	Time		Quantity	Fat	Protein	Carbs	Fibre	kJ/Cal
Breakfast 1 2 3 4 5 ○ ○ ○ ○ ○ HUNGER SCALE								
Mid-morning ○ ○ ○ ○ ○								
Lunch 1 2 3 4 5 ○ ○ ○ ○ ○ HUNGER SCALE								
Mid-afternoon ○ ○ ○ ○ ○								
Dinner 1 2 3 4 5 ○ ○ ○ ○ ○ HUNGER SCALE								
Evening ○ ○ ○ ○ ○								

Coffees/teas   Fluid intake ⛆⛆⛆⛆⛆⛆⛆⛆⛆⛆   Daily totals

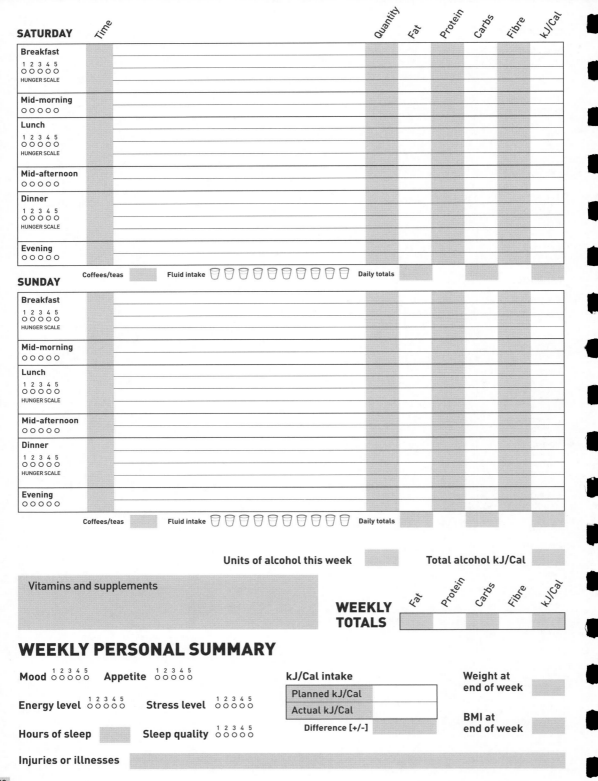

SATURDAY

	Time		Quantity	Fat	Protein	Carbs	Fibre	kJ/Cal
Breakfast 1 2 3 4 5 ○○○○○ HUNGER SCALE								
Mid-morning ○○○○○								
Lunch 1 2 3 4 5 ○○○○○ HUNGER SCALE								
Mid-afternoon ○○○○○								
Dinner 1 2 3 4 5 ○○○○○ HUNGER SCALE								
Evening ○○○○○								

Coffees/teas ▭ Fluid intake ⊔⊔⊔⊔⊔⊔⊔⊔⊔⊔ Daily totals

SUNDAY

	Time		Quantity	Fat	Protein	Carbs	Fibre	kJ/Cal
Breakfast 1 2 3 4 5 ○○○○○ HUNGER SCALE								
Mid-morning ○○○○○								
Lunch 1 2 3 4 5 ○○○○○ HUNGER SCALE								
Mid-afternoon ○○○○○								
Dinner 1 2 3 4 5 ○○○○○ HUNGER SCALE								
Evening ○○○○○								

Coffees/teas ▭ Fluid intake ⊔⊔⊔⊔⊔⊔⊔⊔⊔⊔ Daily totals

Units of alcohol this week ▭   Total alcohol kJ/Cal

Vitamins and supplements

WEEKLY TOTALS

Fat	Protein	Carbs	Fibre	kJ/Cal

WEEKLY PERSONAL SUMMARY

Mood 1 2 3 4 5 ○○○○○   **Appetite** 1 2 3 4 5 ○○○○○

Energy level 1 2 3 4 5 ○○○○○   **Stress level** 1 2 3 4 5 ○○○○○

Hours of sleep ▭   **Sleep quality** 1 2 3 4 5 ○○○○○

kJ/Cal intake

Planned kJ/Cal	
Actual kJ/Cal	
Difference [+/-]	

Weight at end of week

BMI at end of week

Injuries or illnesses

220

EXERCISE DIARY

STRENGTH TRAINING

Exercise	Focus area	SET 1 Reps	SET 1 Weight	SET 2 Reps	SET 2 Weight	SET 3 Reps	SET 3 Weight	SET4 Reps	SET4 Weight	Equipment	Ease

CARDIO TRAINING

Exercise	Time	Distance	Intensity	Heart rate	Ease	kJ/Cal burnt

Total kJ/Cal burnt

INCIDENTAL EXERCISE

Day	Activity	Day	Activity

WEEK BEGINNING / /

Weight at start of week

BMI at start of week

Planned kJ/Cal this week

Possible diet-busting occasions this week

Planned exercise sessions this week

	Exercise	Completed [Y/N]
Monday		
Tuesday		
Wednesday		
Thursday		
Friday		
Saturday		
Sunday		

FOOD DIARY

MONDAY

	Time		Quantity	Fat	Protein	Carbs	Fibre	kJ/Cal
Breakfast 1 2 3 4 5 ○○○○○ HUNGER SCALE								
Mid-morning ○○○○○								
Lunch 1 2 3 4 5 ○○○○○ HUNGER SCALE								
Mid-afternoon ○○○○○								
Dinner 1 2 3 4 5 ○○○○○ HUNGER SCALE								
Evening ○○○○○								

Coffees/teas | Fluid intake ☐☐☐☐☐☐☐☐☐☐ | Daily totals

TUESDAY

	Time		Quantity	Fat	Protein	Carbs	Fibre	kJ/Cal
Breakfast 1 2 3 4 5 ○○○○○ HUNGER SCALE								
Mid-morning ○○○○○								
Lunch 1 2 3 4 5 ○○○○○ HUNGER SCALE								
Mid-afternoon ○○○○○								
Dinner 1 2 3 4 5 ○○○○○ HUNGER SCALE								
Evening ○○○○○								

Coffees/teas | Fluid intake ☐☐☐☐☐☐☐☐☐☐ | Daily totals

WEDNESDAY

	Time		Quantity	Fat	Protein	Carbs	Fibre	kJ/Cal
Breakfast 1 2 3 4 5 ○ ○ ○ ○ ○ HUNGER SCALE								
Mid-morning ○ ○ ○ ○ ○								
Lunch 1 2 3 4 5 ○ ○ ○ ○ ○ HUNGER SCALE								
Mid-afternoon ○ ○ ○ ○ ○								
Dinner 1 2 3 4 5 ○ ○ ○ ○ ○ HUNGER SCALE								
Evening ○ ○ ○ ○ ○								

Coffees/teas ▢   Fluid intake ▽▽▽▽▽▽▽▽▽▽   Daily totals

THURSDAY

	Time		Quantity	Fat	Protein	Carbs	Fibre	kJ/Cal
Breakfast 1 2 3 4 5 ○ ○ ○ ○ ○ HUNGER SCALE								
Mid-morning ○ ○ ○ ○ ○								
Lunch 1 2 3 4 5 ○ ○ ○ ○ ○ HUNGER SCALE								
Mid-afternoon ○ ○ ○ ○ ○								
Dinner 1 2 3 4 5 ○ ○ ○ ○ ○ HUNGER SCALE								
Evening ○ ○ ○ ○ ○								

Coffees/teas ▢   Fluid intake ▽▽▽▽▽▽▽▽▽▽   Daily totals

FRIDAY

	Time		Quantity	Fat	Protein	Carbs	Fibre	kJ/Cal
Breakfast 1 2 3 4 5 ○ ○ ○ ○ ○ HUNGER SCALE								
Mid-morning ○ ○ ○ ○ ○								
Lunch 1 2 3 4 5 ○ ○ ○ ○ ○ HUNGER SCALE								
Mid-afternoon ○ ○ ○ ○ ○								
Dinner 1 2 3 4 5 ○ ○ ○ ○ ○ HUNGER SCALE								
Evening ○ ○ ○ ○ ○								

Coffees/teas ▢   Fluid intake ▽▽▽▽▽▽▽▽▽▽   Daily totals

SATURDAY

	Time		Quantity	Fat	Protein	Carbs	Fibre	kJ/Cal
Breakfast 1 2 3 4 5 ○ ○ ○ ○ ○ HUNGER SCALE								
Mid-morning ○ ○ ○ ○ ○								
Lunch 1 2 3 4 5 ○ ○ ○ ○ ○ HUNGER SCALE								
Mid-afternoon ○ ○ ○ ○ ○								
Dinner 1 2 3 4 5 ○ ○ ○ ○ ○ HUNGER SCALE								
Evening ○ ○ ○ ○ ○								

Coffees/teas ▢   Fluid intake ⊔⊔⊔⊔⊔⊔⊔⊔⊔⊔   Daily totals

SUNDAY

	Time		Quantity	Fat	Protein	Carbs	Fibre	kJ/Cal
Breakfast 1 2 3 4 5 ○ ○ ○ ○ ○ HUNGER SCALE								
Mid-morning ○ ○ ○ ○ ○								
Lunch 1 2 3 4 5 ○ ○ ○ ○ ○ HUNGER SCALE								
Mid-afternoon ○ ○ ○ ○ ○								
Dinner 1 2 3 4 5 ○ ○ ○ ○ ○ HUNGER SCALE								
Evening ○ ○ ○ ○ ○								

Coffees/teas ▢   Fluid intake ⊔⊔⊔⊔⊔⊔⊔⊔⊔⊔   Daily totals

Units of alcohol this week ▢   Total alcohol kJ/Cal ▢

Vitamins and supplements

WEEKLY TOTALS	Fat	Protein	Carbs	Fibre	kJ/Cal

WEEKLY PERSONAL SUMMARY

Mood 1 2 3 4 5 ○ ○ ○ ○ ○   **Appetite** 1 2 3 4 5 ○ ○ ○ ○ ○

Energy level 1 2 3 4 5 ○ ○ ○ ○ ○   **Stress level** 1 2 3 4 5 ○ ○ ○ ○ ○

Hours of sleep ▢   **Sleep quality** 1 2 3 4 5 ○ ○ ○ ○ ○

kJ/Cal intake

Planned kJ/Cal	
Actual kJ/Cal	
Difference [+/-]	

Weight at end of week ▢

BMI at end of week ▢

Injuries or illnesses

224

EXERCISE DIARY

STRENGTH TRAINING		SET 1		SET 2		SET 3		SET 4			
Exercise	Focus area	Reps	Weight	Reps	Weight	Reps	Weight	Reps	Weight	Equipment	Ease

CARDIO TRAINING

Exercise	Time	Distance	Intensity	Heart rate	Ease	kJ/Cal burnt

Total kJ/Cal burnt

INCIDENTAL EXERCISE

Day	Activity	Day	Activity

MONTHLY SUMMARY

MONTH 1   DATE   /   /   AGE [   ]   HEIGHT [   ]

AVERAGE DAILY DIETARY RESULTS

Total your daily dietary results and divide by the number of days in the month to get your daily average.

Fat intake

Goal	
Result	

Difference [+/-]

Protein intake

Goal	
Result	

Difference [+/-]

Carbs intake

Goal	
Result	

Difference [+/-]

Fibre intake

Goal	
Result	

Difference [+/-]

kJ/Cal intake

Goal	
Result	

Difference [+/-]

Add up your daily results (weekly for alcohol) to get your monthly total.

Average daily coffee/teas [   ]

Average daily fluid intake [   ]

Average weekly units of alcohol [   ]

PHYSICAL MEASUREMENTS

LAST MTH'S GOAL		THIS MTH'S RESULT
	Weight	
	BMI	
	Active heart rate	
	Resting heart rate	
	Recovery time	
	Chest	
	Waist	
	Hips	
	Neck	
	Shoulders	
	Right upper arm	
	Left upper arm	
	Right forearm	
	Left forearm	
	Right thigh	
	Left thigh	
	Right calf	
	Left calf	

Place this month's photo here

Add up your weekly planned exercise sessions to get your monthly total.

Number of planned exercise sessions this month [   ]

Number of completed exercise sessions this month [   ]

MONTHLY PERSONAL SUMMARY

Total your weekly results and divide by the number of weeks to get your average.

Average monthly mood 1 2 3 4 5 ○○○○○	**Average monthly appetite** 1 2 3 4 5 ○○○○○	**Average monthly energy level** 1 2 3 4 5 ○○○○○
Average monthly stress level 1 2 3 4 5 ○○○○○	**Average weekly hours of sleep**	**Average monthly sleep quality** 1 2 3 4 5 ○○○○○

NEXT MONTH'S GOALS

AVERAGE DAILY DIETARY GOALS

	NEXT MTH'S GOAL
Fat	
Protein	
Carbs	
Fibre	

	NEXT MTH'S GOAL
kJ/Cal	
Daily fluid intake	
Daily coffee/tea intake	
Weekly alcohol intake	

PHYSICAL MEASUREMENT GOALS

	NEXT MTH'S GOAL
Weight	
BMI	
Active heart rate	
Resting heart rate	
Recovery time	
Chest	
Waist	
Hips	
Neck	

	NEXT MTH'S GOAL
Shoulders	
Right upper arm	
Left upper arm	
Right forearm	
Left forearm	
Right thigh	
Left thigh	
Right calf	
Left calf	

MY PERSONAL GOALS THIS MONTH

MONTHLY SUMMARY

MONTH 2   DATE   /   /   AGE   HEIGHT

AVERAGE DAILY DIETARY RESULTS

Total your daily dietary results and divide by the number of days in the month to get your daily average.

Fat intake

Goal	
Result	

Difference [+/-]

Protein intake

Goal	
Result	

Difference [+/-]

Carbs intake

Goal	
Result	

Difference [+/-]

Fibre intake

Goal	
Result	

Difference [+/-]

kJ/Cal intake

Goal	
Result	

Difference [+/-]

Add up your daily results (weekly for alcohol) to get your monthly total.

Average daily coffee/teas

Average daily fluid intake

Average weekly units of alcohol

PHYSICAL MEASUREMENTS

LAST MTH'S GOAL		THIS MTH'S RESULT
	Weight	
	BMI	
	Active heart rate	
	Resting heart rate	
	Recovery time	
	Chest	
	Waist	
	Hips	
	Neck	
	Shoulders	
	Right upper arm	
	Left upper arm	
	Right forearm	
	Left forearm	
	Right thigh	
	Left thigh	
	Right calf	
	Left calf	

Place this month's photo here

Add up your weekly planned exercise sessions to get your monthly total.

Number of planned exercise sessions this month

Number of completed exercise sessions this month

MONTHLY PERSONAL SUMMARY

Total your weekly results and divide by the number of weeks to get your average.

| Average monthly mood | 1 2 3 4 5 ○○○○○ | Average monthly appetite | 1 2 3 4 5 ○○○○○ | Average monthly energy level | 1 2 3 4 5 ○○○○○ |

| Average monthly stress level | 1 2 3 4 5 ○○○○○ | Average weekly hours of sleep | | Average monthly sleep quality | 1 2 3 4 5 ○○○○○ |

NEXT MONTH'S GOALS

AVERAGE DAILY DIETARY GOALS

	NEXT MTH'S GOAL
Fat	
Protein	
Carbs	
Fibre	

	NEXT MTH'S GOAL
kJ/Cal	
Daily fluid intake	
Daily coffee/tea intake	
Weekly alcohol intake	

PHYSICAL MEASUREMENT GOALS

	NEXT MTH'S GOAL
Weight	
BMI	
Active heart rate	
Resting heart rate	
Recovery time	
Chest	
Waist	
Hips	
Neck	

	NEXT MTH'S GOAL
Shoulders	
Right upper arm	
Left upper arm	
Right forearm	
Left forearm	
Right thigh	
Left thigh	
Right calf	
Left calf	

MY PERSONAL GOALS THIS MONTH

MONTHLY SUMMARY

MONTH 3   DATE [ ] / [ ] / [ ]   AGE [   ]   HEIGHT [   ]

AVERAGE DAILY DIETARY RESULTS

Total your daily dietary results and divide by the number of days in the month to get your daily average.

Fat intake

Goal	
Result	

Difference [+/-] [   ]

Protein intake

Goal	
Result	

Difference [+/-] [   ]

Carbs intake

Goal	
Result	

Difference [+/-] [   ]

Fibre intake

Goal	
Result	

Difference [+/-] [   ]

kJ/Cal intake

Goal	
Result	

Difference [+/-] [   ]

Add up your daily results (weekly for alcohol) to get your monthly total.

Average daily coffee/teas [   ]

Average daily fluid intake [   ]

Average weekly units of alcohol [   ]

PHYSICAL MEASUREMENTS

LAST MTH'S GOAL		THIS MTH'S RESULT
	Weight	
	BMI	
	Active heart rate	
	Resting heart rate	
	Recovery time	
	Chest	
	Waist	
	Hips	
	Neck	
	Shoulders	
	Right upper arm	
	Left upper arm	
	Right forearm	
	Left forearm	
	Right thigh	
	Left thigh	
	Right calf	
	Left calf	

Place this month's photo here

Add up your weekly planned exercise sessions to get your monthly total.

Number of planned exercise sessions this month [   ]

Number of completed exercise sessions this month [   ]

MONTHLY PERSONAL SUMMARY

Total your weekly results and divide by the number of weeks to get your average.

Average monthly mood 1 2 3 4 5 ○○○○○

Average monthly appetite 1 2 3 4 5 ○○○○○

Average monthly energy level 1 2 3 4 5 ○○○○○

Average monthly stress level 1 2 3 4 5 ○○○○○

Average weekly hours of sleep

Average monthly sleep quality 1 2 3 4 5 ○○○○○

NEXT MONTH'S GOALS

AVERAGE DAILY DIETARY GOALS

	NEXT MTH'S GOAL
Fat	
Protein	
Carbs	
Fibre	

	NEXT MTH'S GOAL
kJ/Cal	
Daily fluid intake	
Daily coffee/tea intake	
Weekly alcohol intake	

PHYSICAL MEASUREMENT GOALS

	NEXT MTH'S GOAL
Weight	
BMI	
Active heart rate	
Resting heart rate	
Recovery time	
Chest	
Waist	
Hips	
Neck	

	NEXT MTH'S GOAL
Shoulders	
Right upper arm	
Left upper arm	
Right forearm	
Left forearm	
Right thigh	
Left thigh	
Right calf	
Left calf	

MY PERSONAL GOALS THIS MONTH

MONTHLY SUMMARY

MONTH 4   DATE [/ /]   AGE [ ]   HEIGHT [ ]

AVERAGE DAILY DIETARY RESULTS

Total your daily dietary results and divide by the number of days in the month to get your daily average.

Fat intake

Goal	
Result	

Difference [+/-]

Protein intake

Goal	
Result	

Difference [+/-]

Carbs intake

Goal	
Result	

Difference [+/-]

Fibre intake

Goal	
Result	

Difference [+/-]

kJ/Cal intake

Goal	
Result	

Difference [+/-]

Add up your daily results (weekly for alcohol) to get your monthly total.

Average daily coffee/teas [ ]

Average daily fluid intake [ ]

Average weekly units of alcohol [ ]

PHYSICAL MEASUREMENTS

LAST MTH'S GOAL		THIS MTH'S RESULT
	Weight	
	BMI	
	Active heart rate	
	Resting heart rate	
	Recovery time	
	Chest	
	Waist	
	Hips	
	Neck	
	Shoulders	
	Right upper arm	
	Left upper arm	
	Right forearm	
	Left forearm	
	Right thigh	
	Left thigh	
	Right calf	
	Left calf	

Place this month's photo here

Add up your weekly planned exercise sessions to get your monthly total.

Number of planned exercise sessions this month [ ]

Number of completed exercise sessions this month [ ]

232

MONTHLY PERSONAL SUMMARY

Total your weekly results and divide by the number of weeks to get your average.

Average monthly mood 1 2 3 4 5 ○○○○○

Average monthly appetite 1 2 3 4 5 ○○○○○

Average monthly energy level 1 2 3 4 5 ○○○○○

Average monthly stress level 1 2 3 4 5 ○○○○○

Average weekly hours of sleep

Average monthly sleep quality 1 2 3 4 5 ○○○○○

NEXT MONTH'S GOALS

AVERAGE DAILY DIETARY GOALS

	NEXT MTH'S GOAL
Fat	
Protein	
Carbs	
Fibre	

	NEXT MTH'S GOAL
kJ/Cal	
Daily fluid intake	
Daily coffee/tea intake	
Weekly alcohol intake	

PHYSICAL MEASUREMENT GOALS

	NEXT MTH'S GOAL
Weight	
BMI	
Active heart rate	
Resting heart rate	
Recovery time	
Chest	
Waist	
Hips	
Neck	

	NEXT MTH'S GOAL
Shoulders	
Right upper arm	
Left upper arm	
Right forearm	
Left forearm	
Right thigh	
Left thigh	
Right calf	
Left calf	

MY PERSONAL GOALS THIS MONTH

MONTHLY SUMMARY

MONTH 5   DATE ___ / ___ / ___   AGE _____   HEIGHT _____

AVERAGE DAILY DIETARY RESULTS

Total your daily dietary results and divide by the number of days in the month to get your daily average.

Fat intake

Goal	
Result	

Difference [+/-]

Protein intake

Goal	
Result	

Difference [+/-]

Carbs intake

Goal	
Result	

Difference [+/-]

Fibre intake

Goal	
Result	

Difference [+/-]

kJ/Cal intake

Goal	
Result	

Difference [+/-]

Add up your daily results (weekly for alcohol) to get your monthly total.

Average daily coffee/teas _____

Average daily fluid intake _____

Average weekly units of alcohol _____

PHYSICAL MEASUREMENTS

LAST MTH'S GOAL		THIS MTH'S RESULT
	Weight	
	BMI	
	Active heart rate	
	Resting heart rate	
	Recovery time	
	Chest	
	Waist	
	Hips	
	Neck	
	Shoulders	
	Right upper arm	
	Left upper arm	
	Right forearm	
	Left forearm	
	Right thigh	
	Left thigh	
	Right calf	
	Left calf	

Place this month's photo here

Add up your weekly planned exercise sessions to get your monthly total.

Number of planned exercise sessions this month _____

Number of completed exercise sessions this month _____

MONTHLY PERSONAL SUMMARY

Total your weekly results and divide by the number of weeks to get your average.

Average monthly mood 1 2 3 4 5 ○○○○○	**Average monthly appetite** 1 2 3 4 5 ○○○○○	**Average monthly energy level** 1 2 3 4 5 ○○○○○	
Average monthly stress level 1 2 3 4 5 ○○○○○	**Average weekly hours of sleep**	**Average monthly sleep quality** 1 2 3 4 5 ○○○○○	

NEXT MONTH'S GOALS

AVERAGE DAILY DIETARY GOALS

	NEXT MTH'S GOAL
Fat	
Protein	
Carbs	
Fibre	

	NEXT MTH'S GOAL
kJ/Cal	
Daily fluid intake	
Daily coffee/tea intake	
Weekly alcohol intake	

PHYSICAL MEASUREMENT GOALS

	NEXT MTH'S GOAL
Weight	
BMI	
Active heart rate	
Resting heart rate	
Recovery time	
Chest	
Waist	
Hips	
Neck	

	NEXT MTH'S GOAL
Shoulders	
Right upper arm	
Left upper arm	
Right forearm	
Left forearm	
Right thigh	
Left thigh	
Right calf	
Left calf	

MY PERSONAL GOALS THIS MONTH

MONTHLY SUMMARY

MONTH 6   DATE   /   /   AGE   HEIGHT

AVERAGE DAILY DIETARY RESULTS

Total your daily dietary results and divide by the number of days in the month to get your daily average.

Fat intake

Goal	
Result	

Difference [+/-]

Protein intake

Goal	
Result	

Difference [+/-]

Carbs intake

Goal	
Result	

Difference [+/-]

Fibre intake

Goal	
Result	

Difference [+/-]

kJ/Cal intake

Goal	
Result	

Difference [+/-]

Add up your daily results (weekly for alcohol) to get your monthly total.

Average daily coffee/teas

Average daily fluid intake

Average weekly units of alcohol

PHYSICAL MEASUREMENTS

LAST MTH'S GOAL		THIS MTH'S RESULT
	Weight	
	BMI	
	Active heart rate	
	Resting heart rate	
	Recovery time	
	Chest	
	Waist	
	Hips	
	Neck	
	Shoulders	
	Right upper arm	
	Left upper arm	
	Right forearm	
	Left forearm	
	Right thigh	
	Left thigh	
	Right calf	
	Left calf	

Place this month's photo here

Add up your weekly planned exercise sessions to get your monthly total.

Number of planned exercise sessions this month

Number of completed exercise sessions this month

MONTHLY PERSONAL SUMMARY

Total your weekly results and divide by the number of weeks to get your average.

Average monthly mood 1 2 3 4 5 ○ ○ ○ ○ ○	**Average monthly appetite** 1 2 3 4 5 ○ ○ ○ ○ ○
Average monthly energy level 1 2 3 4 5 ○ ○ ○ ○ ○	

Average monthly stress level 1 2 3 4 5 ○ ○ ○ ○ ○	**Average weekly hours of sleep**
Average monthly sleep quality 1 2 3 4 5 ○ ○ ○ ○ ○	

NEXT MONTH'S GOALS

AVERAGE DAILY DIETARY GOALS

	NEXT MTH'S GOAL
Fat	
Protein	
Carbs	
Fibre	

	NEXT MTH'S GOAL
kJ/Cal	
Daily fluid intake	
Daily coffee/tea intake	
Weekly alcohol intake	

PHYSICAL MEASUREMENT GOALS

	NEXT MTH'S GOAL
Weight	
BMI	
Active heart rate	
Resting heart rate	
Recovery time	
Chest	
Waist	
Hips	
Neck	

	NEXT MTH'S GOAL
Shoulders	
Right upper arm	
Left upper arm	
Right forearm	
Left forearm	
Right thigh	
Left thigh	
Right calf	
Left calf	

MY PERSONAL GOALS THIS MONTH

MONTHLY SUMMARY

MONTH 7   **DATE** ___ / ___ / ___   **AGE** _____   **HEIGHT** _____

AVERAGE DAILY DIETARY RESULTS

Total your daily dietary results and divide by the number of days in the month to get your daily average.

Fat intake

Goal	
Result	

Difference [+/-]

Protein intake

Goal	
Result	

Difference [+/-]

Carbs intake

Goal	
Result	

Difference [+/-]

Fibre intake

Goal	
Result	

Difference [+/-]

kJ/Cal intake

Goal	
Result	

Difference [+/-]

Add up your daily results (weekly for alcohol) to get your monthly total.

Average daily coffee/teas _____

Average daily fluid intake _____

Average weekly units of alcohol _____

PHYSICAL MEASUREMENTS

LAST MTH'S GOAL		THIS MTH'S RESULT
	Weight	
	BMI	
	Active heart rate	
	Resting heart rate	
	Recovery time	
	Chest	
	Waist	
	Hips	
	Neck	
	Shoulders	
	Right upper arm	
	Left upper arm	
	Right forearm	
	Left forearm	
	Right thigh	
	Left thigh	
	Right calf	
	Left calf	

Place this month's photo here

Add up your weekly planned exercise sessions to get your monthly total.

Number of planned exercise sessions this month _____

Number of completed exercise sessions this month _____

MONTHLY PERSONAL SUMMARY

Total your weekly results and divide by the number of weeks to get your average.

Average monthly mood 1 2 3 4 5 ○○○○○

Average monthly appetite 1 2 3 4 5 ○○○○○

Average monthly energy level 1 2 3 4 5 ○○○○○

Average monthly stress level 1 2 3 4 5 ○○○○○

Average weekly hours of sleep

Average monthly sleep quality 1 2 3 4 5 ○○○○○

NEXT MONTH'S GOALS

AVERAGE DAILY DIETARY GOALS

	NEXT MTH'S GOAL
Fat	
Protein	
Carbs	
Fibre	

	NEXT MTH'S GOAL
kJ/Cal	
Daily fluid intake	
Daily coffee/tea intake	
Weekly alcohol intake	

PHYSICAL MEASUREMENT GOALS

	NEXT MTH'S GOAL
Weight	
BMI	
Active heart rate	
Resting heart rate	
Recovery time	
Chest	
Waist	
Hips	
Neck	

	NEXT MTH'S GOAL
Shoulders	
Right upper arm	
Left upper arm	
Right forearm	
Left forearm	
Right thigh	
Left thigh	
Right calf	
Left calf	

MY PERSONAL GOALS THIS MONTH

MONTHLY SUMMARY

MONTH 8   **DATE**   /   /   **AGE**   **HEIGHT**

AVERAGE DAILY DIETARY RESULTS

Total your daily dietary results and divide by the number of days in the month to get your daily average.

Fat intake

Goal	
Result	

Difference [+/-]

Protein intake

Goal	
Result	

Difference [+/-]

Carbs intake

Goal	
Result	

Difference [+/-]

Fibre intake

Goal	
Result	

Difference [+/-]

kJ/Cal intake

Goal	
Result	

Difference [+/-]

Add up your daily results (weekly for alcohol) to get your monthly total.

Average daily coffee/teas

Average daily fluid intake

Average weekly units of alcohol

PHYSICAL MEASUREMENTS

LAST MTH'S GOAL		THIS MTH'S RESULT
	Weight	
	BMI	
	Active heart rate	
	Resting heart rate	
	Recovery time	
	Chest	
	Waist	
	Hips	
	Neck	
	Shoulders	
	Right upper arm	
	Left upper arm	
	Right forearm	
	Left forearm	
	Right thigh	
	Left thigh	
	Right calf	
	Left calf	

Place this month's photo here

Add up your weekly planned exercise sessions to get your monthly total.

Number of planned exercise sessions this month

Number of completed exercise sessions this month

MONTHLY PERSONAL SUMMARY

Total your weekly results and divide by the number of weeks to get your average.

	1 2 3 4 5		1 2 3 4 5		1 2 3 4 5
Average monthly mood	○○○○○	**Average monthly appetite**	○○○○○	**Average monthly energy level**	○○○○○
Average monthly stress level	○○○○○	**Average weekly hours of sleep**		**Average monthly sleep quality**	○○○○○

NEXT MONTH'S GOALS

AVERAGE DAILY DIETARY GOALS

	NEXT MTH'S GOAL		NEXT MTH'S GOAL
Fat		kJ/Cal	
Protein		Daily fluid intake	
Carbs		Daily coffee/tea intake	
Fibre		Weekly alcohol intake	

PHYSICAL MEASUREMENT GOALS

	NEXT MTH'S GOAL		NEXT MTH'S GOAL
Weight		Shoulders	
BMI		Right upper arm	
Active heart rate		Left upper arm	
Resting heart rate		Right forearm	
Recovery time		Left forearm	
Chest		Right thigh	
Waist		Left thigh	
Hips		Right calf	
Neck		Left calf	

MY PERSONAL GOALS THIS MONTH

MONTHLY SUMMARY

MONTH 9   **DATE** / /   **AGE**   **HEIGHT**

AVERAGE DAILY DIETARY RESULTS

Total your daily dietary results and divide by the number of days in the month to get your daily average.

Fat intake

Goal	
Result	

Difference [+/-]

Protein intake

Goal	
Result	

Difference [+/-]

Carbs intake

Goal	
Result	

Difference [+/-]

Fibre intake

Goal	
Result	

Difference [+/-]

kJ/Cal intake

Goal	
Result	

Difference [+/-]

Add up your daily results (weekly for alcohol) to get your monthly total.

Average daily coffee/teas

Average daily fluid intake

Average weekly units of alcohol

PHYSICAL MEASUREMENTS

LAST MTH'S GOAL		THIS MTH'S RESULT
	Weight	
	BMI	
	Active heart rate	
	Resting heart rate	
	Recovery time	
	Chest	
	Waist	
	Hips	
	Neck	
	Shoulders	
	Right upper arm	
	Left upper arm	
	Right forearm	
	Left forearm	
	Right thigh	
	Left thigh	
	Right calf	
	Left calf	

Place this month's photo here

Add up your weekly planned exercise sessions to get your monthly total.

Number of planned exercise sessions this month

Number of completed exercise sessions this month

MONTHLY PERSONAL SUMMARY

Total your weekly results and divide by the number of weeks to get your average.

Average monthly mood 1 2 3 4 5 ○○○○○	**Average monthly appetite** 1 2 3 4 5 ○○○○○	**Average monthly energy level** 1 2 3 4 5 ○○○○○
Average monthly stress level 1 2 3 4 5 ○○○○○	**Average weekly hours of sleep**	**Average monthly sleep quality** 1 2 3 4 5 ○○○○○

NEXT MONTH'S GOALS

AVERAGE DAILY DIETARY GOALS

	NEXT MTH'S GOAL
Fat	
Protein	
Carbs	
Fibre	

	NEXT MTH'S GOAL
kJ/Cal	
Daily fluid intake	
Daily coffee/tea intake	
Weekly alcohol intake	

PHYSICAL MEASUREMENT GOALS

	NEXT MTH'S GOAL
Weight	
BMI	
Active heart rate	
Resting heart rate	
Recovery time	
Chest	
Waist	
Hips	
Neck	

	NEXT MTH'S GOAL
Shoulders	
Right upper arm	
Left upper arm	
Right forearm	
Left forearm	
Right thigh	
Left thigh	
Right calf	
Left calf	

MY PERSONAL GOALS THIS MONTH

MONTHLY SUMMARY

MONTH 10   DATE ___ / ___ / ___   AGE _____   HEIGHT _____

AVERAGE DAILY DIETARY RESULTS

Total your daily dietary results and divide by the number of days in the month to get your daily average.

Fat intake

Goal	
Result	

Difference [+/-]

Protein intake

Goal	
Result	

Difference [+/-]

Carbs intake

Goal	
Result	

Difference [+/-]

Fibre intake

Goal	
Result	

Difference [+/-]

kJ/Cal intake

Goal	
Result	

Difference [+/-]

Add up your daily results (weekly for alcohol) to get your monthly total.

Average daily coffee/teas _____

Average daily fluid intake _____

Average weekly units of alcohol _____

PHYSICAL MEASUREMENTS

LAST MTH'S GOAL		THIS MTH'S RESULT
	Weight	
	BMI	
	Active heart rate	
	Resting heart rate	
	Recovery time	
	Chest	
	Waist	
	Hips	
	Neck	
	Shoulders	
	Right upper arm	
	Left upper arm	
	Right forearm	
	Left forearm	
	Right thigh	
	Left thigh	
	Right calf	
	Left calf	

Place this month's photo here

Add up your weekly planned exercise sessions to get your monthly total.

Number of planned exercise sessions this month _____

Number of completed exercise sessions this month _____

MONTHLY PERSONAL SUMMARY

Total your weekly results and divide by the number of weeks to get your average.

	1 2 3 4 5		1 2 3 4 5		1 2 3 4 5
Average monthly mood	○ ○ ○ ○ ○	**Average monthly appetite**	○ ○ ○ ○ ○	**Average monthly energy level**	○ ○ ○ ○ ○
Average monthly stress level	○ ○ ○ ○ ○	**Average weekly hours of sleep**		**Average monthly sleep quality**	○ ○ ○ ○ ○

NEXT MONTH'S GOALS

AVERAGE DAILY DIETARY GOALS

	NEXT MTH'S GOAL
Fat	
Protein	
Carbs	
Fibre	

	NEXT MTH'S GOAL
kJ/Cal	
Daily fluid intake	
Daily coffee/tea intake	
Weekly alcohol intake	

PHYSICAL MEASUREMENT GOALS

	NEXT MTH'S GOAL
Weight	
BMI	
Active heart rate	
Resting heart rate	
Recovery time	
Chest	
Waist	
Hips	
Neck	

	NEXT MTH'S GOAL
Shoulders	
Right upper arm	
Left upper arm	
Right forearm	
Left forearm	
Right thigh	
Left thigh	
Right calf	
Left calf	

MY PERSONAL GOALS THIS MONTH

MONTHLY SUMMARY

MONTH 11   DATE   /   /   AGE   HEIGHT

AVERAGE DAILY DIETARY RESULTS

Total your daily dietary results and divide by the number of days in the month to get your daily average.

Fat intake

Goal	
Result	

Difference [+/-]

Protein intake

Goal	
Result	

Difference [+/-]

Carbs intake

Goal	
Result	

Difference [+/-]

Fibre intake

Goal	
Result	

Difference [+/-]

kJ/Cal intake

Goal	
Result	

Difference [+/-]

Add up your daily results (weekly for alcohol) to get your monthly total.

Average daily coffee/teas

Average daily fluid intake

Average weekly units of alcohol

PHYSICAL MEASUREMENTS

LAST MTH'S GOAL		THIS MTH'S RESULT
	Weight	
	BMI	
	Active heart rate	
	Resting heart rate	
	Recovery time	
	Chest	
	Waist	
	Hips	
	Neck	
	Shoulders	
	Right upper arm	
	Left upper arm	
	Right forearm	
	Left forearm	
	Right thigh	
	Left thigh	
	Right calf	
	Left calf	

Place this month's photo here

Add up your weekly planned exercise sessions to get your monthly total.

Number of planned exercise sessions this month

Number of completed exercise sessions this month

MONTHLY PERSONAL SUMMARY

Total your weekly results and divide by the number of weeks to get your average.

Average monthly mood 1 2 3 4 5 ○○○○○	**Average monthly appetite** 1 2 3 4 5 ○○○○○	**Average monthly energy level** 1 2 3 4 5 ○○○○○
Average monthly stress level 1 2 3 4 5 ○○○○○	**Average weekly hours of sleep**	**Average monthly sleep quality** 1 2 3 4 5 ○○○○○

NEXT MONTH'S GOALS

AVERAGE DAILY DIETARY GOALS

	NEXT MTH'S GOAL
Fat	
Protein	
Carbs	
Fibre	

	NEXT MTH'S GOAL
kJ/Cal	
Daily fluid intake	
Daily coffee/tea intake	
Weekly alcohol intake	

PHYSICAL MEASUREMENT GOALS

	NEXT MTH'S GOAL
Weight	
BMI	
Active heart rate	
Resting heart rate	
Recovery time	
Chest	
Waist	
Hips	
Neck	

	NEXT MTH'S GOAL
Shoulders	
Right upper arm	
Left upper arm	
Right forearm	
Left forearm	
Right thigh	
Left thigh	
Right calf	
Left calf	

MY PERSONAL GOALS THIS MONTH

MONTHLY SUMMARY

MONTH 12   DATE ___/___/___   AGE [___]   HEIGHT [___]

AVERAGE DAILY DIETARY RESULTS

Total your daily dietary results and divide by the number of days in the month to get your daily average.

Fat intake

Goal	
Result	

Difference [+/-]

Protein intake

Goal	
Result	

Difference [+/-]

Carbs intake

Goal	
Result	

Difference [+/-]

Fibre intake

Goal	
Result	

Difference [+/-]

kJ/Cal intake

Goal	
Result	

Difference [+/-]

Add up your daily results (weekly for alcohol) to get your monthly total.

Average daily coffee/teas [___]

Average daily fluid intake [___]

Average weekly units of alcohol [___]

PHYSICAL MEASUREMENTS

LAST MTH'S GOAL		THIS MTH'S RESULT
	Weight	
	BMI	
	Active heart rate	
	Resting heart rate	
	Recovery time	
	Chest	
	Waist	
	Hips	
	Neck	
	Shoulders	
	Right upper arm	
	Left upper arm	
	Right forearm	
	Left forearm	
	Right thigh	
	Left thigh	
	Right calf	
	Left calf	

Place this month's photo here

Add up your weekly planned exercise sessions to get your monthly total.

Number of planned exercise sessions this month [___]

Number of completed exercise sessions this month [___]

MONTHLY PERSONAL SUMMARY

Total your weekly results and divide by the number of weeks to get your average.

Average monthly mood 1 2 3 4 5 ○○○○○	**Average monthly appetite** 1 2 3 4 5 ○○○○○	**Average monthly energy level** 1 2 3 4 5 ○○○○○
Average monthly stress level 1 2 3 4 5 ○○○○○	**Average weekly hours of sleep**	**Average monthly sleep quality** 1 2 3 4 5 ○○○○○

NEXT MONTH'S GOALS

AVERAGE DAILY DIETARY GOALS

	NEXT MTH'S GOAL
Fat	
Protein	
Carbs	
Fibre	

	NEXT MTH'S GOAL
kJ/Cal	
Daily fluid intake	
Daily coffee/tea intake	
Weekly alcohol intake	

PHYSICAL MEASUREMENT GOALS

	NEXT MTH'S GOAL
Weight	
BMI	
Active heart rate	
Resting heart rate	
Recovery time	
Chest	
Waist	
Hips	
Neck	

	NEXT MTH'S GOAL
Shoulders	
Right upper arm	
Left upper arm	
Right forearm	
Left forearm	
Right thigh	
Left thigh	
Right calf	
Left calf	

MY PERSONAL GOALS THIS MONTH

END-OF-YEAR ASSESSMENT

DATE ____ / ____ / ____   AGE _____   HEIGHT _____

START-OF-YEAR PHYSICAL MEASUREMENT TARGETS		ACTUAL PHYSICAL MEASUREMENT RESULTS		Difference [+/-]
Weight		Weight		
BMI		BMI		
Active heart rate		Active heart rate		
Resting heart rate		Resting heart rate		
Recovery time		Recovery time		
Chest		Chest		
Waist		Waist		
Hips		Hips		
Neck		Neck		
Shoulders		Shoulders		
Right upper arm		Right upper arm		
Left upper arm		Left upper arm		
Right forearm		Right forearm		
Left forearm		Left forearm		
Right thigh		Right thigh		
Left thigh		Left thigh		
Right calf		Right calf		
Left calf		Left calf		

Target clothes size _____   Actual clothes size _____   Difference [+/-] _____

Time how long it takes you to walk 2 km or 1 mile.

Target time _____   Actual time _____   Difference [+/-] _____

Count how many push-ups you can do before you have to stop.

Target number of push-ups _____   Actual number of push-ups _____   Difference [+/-] _____

Count how many sit-ups you can do in 1 minute.

Target number of sit-ups _____   Actual number of sit-ups _____   Difference [+/-] _____

Count how many squats you can do before you have to stop.

Target number of squats _____   Actual number of squats _____   Difference [+/-] _____

Sit on the floor with your legs out straight. Place a ruler on the floor with the centre measurement between your feet. Record how many cm/inches you can stretch up to [-] or beyond [+] your feet.

Target distance [+/-] _____   Actual distance [+/-] _____   Difference [+/-] _____

END-OF-YEAR PERSONAL SUMMARY

Place end-of-year
photo here

Satisfaction with weight   0   5   10

Satisfaction with fitness   0   5   10

Quality of diet   0   5   10

Strength level   0   5   10

Endurance level   0   5   10

Sleep quality   0   5   10

Mood level   0   5   10

Stress level   0   5   10

Energy level   0   5   10

MY PERSONAL SUCCESSES THIS YEAR

MY PERSONAL GOALS FOR NEXT YEAR

YEARLY WEIGHT GRAPH

WEIGHT

150kg
146kg
142kg
138kg
134kg
130kg
126kg
122kg
118kg
114kg
110kg
106kg
102kg
98kg
94kg
90kg
86kg
82kg
78kg
74kg
70kg
66kg
62kg
58kg
54kg
50kg
46kg
42kg
38kg
34kg
30kg

1　2　3　4　5　6　7　8　9　10　11　12　13　14　15　16　17　18　19　20　21　22　23　24　25　26

WEEK

Record your weekly weight and graph your progress throughout the year.

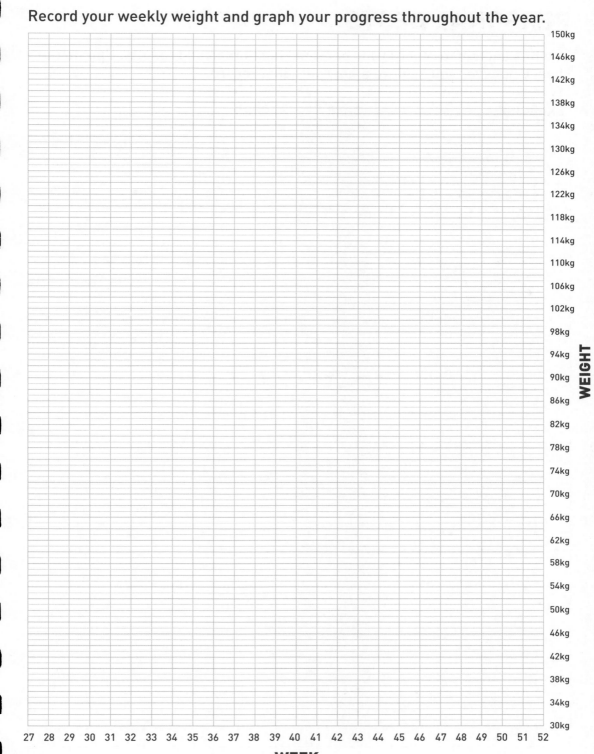

WEIGHT

WEEK

PERSONAL BESTS

Use this section to record your personal best times and results. Update the chart whenever you achieve a new personal record.

EXERCISE	DATE	RECORD

EXERCISE	DATE	RECORD

DIET AND EXERCISE NOTES